KOREAN STUDIES SERIES No. 29

An Introduction to Sasang Constitutional Medicine

Written by Song Il-byung
Translated by Joseph K. Kim &
Huh Mahn-hoi
Edited by Floyd E. Sandoval &
Naomi R. Gelperin

Projected by The Society of Sasang
Constitutional Medicine

Jimoondang International
Edison · Seoul

KOREAN STUDIES SERIES No. 29

An Introduction to Sasang Constitutional Medicine

Jimoondang International
227 Suttons Lane, Edison, NJ 08817 U.S.A.
Phone: (732) 777-9650 Fax: (732) 777-3348
E-mail: jimoondang@yahoo.com
Library of Congress Control Number: 2005920408
ISBN 1-931897-09-3

Published simultaneously in Korea
by Jimoondang
535 Munbal-ri Gyoha-eup Paju-si Gyeonggi-do, 413-832 Korea
Phone: 82-2-743-0227 E-mail: edit@jimoon.co.kr
82-2-743-3192～3 E-mail: sale@jimoon.co.kr
F a x: 82-2-743-3097, 82-2-742-4657
Home page: www.jimoon.co.kr

Translator's Foreword

It is my great pleasure and privilege to have translated Professor Song Il-byung's book *An Introduction to Sasang Constitutional Medicine.* Professor Song spent his lifetime studying, researching, and teaching Sasang Constitutional Medicine (SCM). He is currently the foremost exponent of this system of medicine in Korea. Korea has eleven universities with Eastern medical schools, and there, in each of those schools, is a Department of Sasang Constitutional Medicine. All of the heads of those departments have, at one time, been students of Professor Song.

Currently, SCM is one of seven specialties of Eastern medicine in Korea. It is quite popular in Korea not only among doctors of Eastern medicine, but also within the general public. There are over 50 books on the subject and last year a popular TV drama chronicling the life and times of Dr. Lee Je-ma (1837-1900 AD), the creator of SCM, received rave reviews.

In addition to Korea, the Yanbian Province of northeastern China is home to a large Korean population and several students of Dr. Lee Je-ma have lived and taught in that province. Currently in Yanji, a city near the border of North Korea, there is a research center devoted entirely to the study of SCM. SCM is one of only five minority's medicines officially recognized by the Chinese government. The others are Mongolian, Tibetan, Uygur, and Vietnamese medicines.

Other than the Yanbian Province of China, SCM is not well known outside Korea, particularly since information in English has been scarce. As Professor Song mentioned in his preface, I also hope that with the publication of this translation, SCM will become known throughout the world. Those of you who would like further information on SCM are advised to read two other books in English. One is a translation of the original text of SCM, *Longevity and Life Preservation in Eastern Medicine* (Kyung Hee University Press, 1996: Seoul) by Dr. Choi

Seung-hoon, a professor at Kyung Hee University, and the other is my book, *Compass of Health* (New Page Books, 2001: Franklin Lakes).

In this translation, the names of disease syndromes and most of the formula names for the constitutions were adapted from Dr. Choi Seung-hoon's translation. The translation of Chinese words is presented in pinyin except for the most commonly known terms (i.e. *taichi* and *tao*). Since the physiological actions of various organs differ in SCM from that of western medicine, they were also capitalized to differentiate them from western anatomical organs.

I would like to advise any reader with a medical condition to first consult with their physician prior to following any advice in this book regarding diet, herbal tea, and exercise.

Finally, I would like to thank Professor Song for giving me the opportunity to translate his book. In translating this book, I received invaluable assistance from Dr. Hong Suk-chul, a Professor at Samra University of Oriental Medicine in Los Angeles, and Dr. Huh Mahn-hoi who is the top expert of the body measuring system for diagnosing Sasang constitutions in Korea. Without their help, translating this book would have been an impossible task. I would also like to thank Naomi Gelperin, Licensed Acupuncturist, for her invaluable editing of the entire manuscript.

Joseph K. Kim
Encino, California
April 2004

Preface

In 1894, Dr. Lee Je-ma wrote *Longevity and Life Preservation in Eastern Medicine* (*Dong-ui susebowon*), the foundational text of Sasang Constitutional Medicine (SCM). Although SCM has been around for more than 100 years, until recently it was considered a specialty among the various methods of Eastern medicine. Few eastern medical doctors practiced SCM, and it was not well known among the general populace. Nevertheless, interest in SCM has been increasing over the past several years and I firmly believe that SCM will greatly contribute to increasing the health of many people.

Although there are several reasons for the increased interest in SCM, there are two that are significant. The first is a change in attitude about the benefits and risks of eastern and western medicine. People have begun to move away from having an unconditional faith in western culture and ideology, and have gained a renewed interest in eastern ideology and Eastern medicine. The second reason is that SCM is very accessible to the common people. Anyone can easily use the medicine for health maintenance. SCM is not only curative; it is also a preventative medicine. It is a method of health cultivation as well as a way of life that can show people how to have more enjoyable and healthier lives. It is not an exaggeration to say that a person could learn methods of health cultivation and longevity from SCM with no prior technical knowledge of Eastern medicine. Furthermore, people can also learn methods of wisdom and proper conduct in order to form harmonious personal, social, and professional relationships.

However, even with such a wonderful medicine in our midst, there has been little headway made in terms of its research, development, and popularization. In spite of this, SCM is widely recognized and approved of by many people.

I have two reasons for writing this book. The first is to respond to the increased demand for a book about SCM that is easy to understand. That said I realize that this book may not explain all of the principles of SCM for it is, by nature, a very complicated subject. The other reason is to help correct any misunderstandings that have arisen as a result of the growing interest in SCM. Where did these misunderstandings of SCM begin? Dr. Lee Je-ma was a pragmatist who lived at the end of Chosun dynasty (1392-1910 AD). He completed the formation of Sasang philosophy, which is the reformation of Confucianism. Most of the misunderstandings on the subject have been caused by an acceptance of SCM without a proper understanding of Sasang philosophy.

The ultimate goal of SCM is to view the constitution using the philosophy of the "Golden Mean" or "Middle Path" and to guide the inherently tilted prenatal body to "center" by postnatal efforts. This is the fundamental treatment principle of SCM as well as its method of health cultivation, which varies according to each constitution. It can be accomplished through the proper regulation of the physical body and with environmental adaptations. Moreover, SCM tries to teach people to maintain harmony with all things while maintaining a balance of body and mind.

The recent understanding of SCM is primarily based on the treatment principles of the *Nei Jing* (Yellow Emperor's Classic of Internal Medicine) or theories summarized in the *I Ching* rather than on Sasang philosophy. Because of this, the theory of the Sasang constitutions has been misinterpreted. This book will attempt to point out these misinterpretations.

This book has five chapters with extensive appendices. The first three chapters focus on subjects that can be easily understood and readily applied by anyone. Chapters 4, 5 and the appendices are a bit more technical. This is the result of trying to accommodate to the general public while keeping the essence of SCM intact. It would be beneficial for the reader to first read the information contained in chapters 1, 2 and 3, and apply those principles to their lives and once this is done, come back and read chapters 4 and 5.

Finally, I would like to thank my good friends who

supported my efforts. First of all, I would like to thank Professor Ko Byung-hee who gave me so much invaluable advice. And I cannot forget the efforts of Dr. Park Sung-sik who carefully scrutinized and edited the entire manuscript amidst his busy schedule. I would also like to give my wholehearted appreciation to Mr. Hwang In-sang, who helped me from the planning stages to the actual publication of this book. Finally, I would like to thank the President of Hana Media Publishing, Mr. Chung Ji-suk, who kindly accepted and published the complicated manuscript.

Song Il-byung
In the office of Kyung Hee University Clinic
December 10, 2001

Preface to the English Translation

TCM, known as "syndrome medicine," treats disease through methods of tonification and sedation, which are based on the principle of "supplementing the righteous energy and eliminating pathogenic factors." In contrast, Sasang Constitutional Medicine looks first at the "constitutional self-rectification" of the Sasang constitutions as a method of self-cultivation based on the principle of "cultivating oneself and providing service to others" found in Confucianism. This is then applied as a method of character cultivation and means of disease treatment for the Sasang constitutions.

Dr. Lee Je-ma presented the wisdom of finding the "constitutional self-rectification" within daily life in two ways: self-rectification based on health cultivation and self-rectification based on herbal medicine. He called the former, "the scholarly way" and the latter, "the military way."

In the form of self-rectification that is based on health cultivation, Dr. Lee Je-ma presented methods of "self-rectification by cultivating the Heart or the mind," which is the self-rectification of one's inner nature and emotions, and "self-rectification based on proper knowledge and conduct," which is the self-rectification involved in daily life. He used these two methods as modes of character cultivation and disease prevention for the Sasang constitutions. Additionally, he presented self-rectification based on herbal medicine as a means of disease treatment.

It was through the treatment methods of "the scholarly way" and "the military way" that Dr. Lee Je-ma presented the treatment principles of Sasang Constitutional Medicine. The treatment principles originate from the spirit of "regulation based on the Golden Mean" of Confucianism. I am proud of the development of medical treatment principles based on the new paradigm of the Sasang Constitutional Theory with its background in Confucianism that have been set forth in Korea. I would also like to take this opportunity to express my joy in knowing that the Sasang Constitutional Medicine will become known worldwide with the publication of the English edition of this book.

I'd like to thank Dr. Joseph K. Kim and Dr. Huh Mahn-hoi who translated this Korean edition and Floyd E. Sandoval who edited and reviewed the translated edition in concurrence with the Sasang Executive Committee; Dr. Song Il-byung, Prof. Ko Byung-hee, Prof. Lee Eui-joo, Prof. Lee Soo-kyung, Dr. Huh Mahn-hoi. I cannot forget the first trial and efforts of having translated this book, ahead of Dr. Joseph Kim's translation, with the help of Jung K. Kim, L.Ac., Hoon Cheol Kim, L.Ac., Sun Young Park.

Finally, I'd like to thank the President of Jimoondang Publishing, Mr. Lim, who kindly accepted and published this English translated edition.

Song Il-byung
Head Professor, Department of Sasang Constitutional Medicine
Kyung Hee University, January 2004

Editor's Preface

It is my great pleasure and honor to have edited Professor Song Il-byung's book *An Introduction to Sasang Constitutional Medicine*. I would like to first thank Professor Song for giving me the opportunity to edit his book. I began editing the manuscript after identifying inherent translation irregularities and contradictions.

Great care was given to accurately express the true meaning and philosophy of Dr. Lee Je-ma's Theory of Sasang Constitutional Medicine. Many months were spent reviewing, modifying and correcting editorial and translation changes in concurrence with the Sasang Executive Committee to insure that clarity, accuracy, and objectivity was given the utmost priority. As a result, the readers will receive an accurate comprehensive translation of *An Introduction to Sasang Constitutional Medicine*.

In editing this book, I received invaluable assistance from Dr. Huh Mahn-hoi who is a second generation Sasang Medical doctor, international lecturer, publisher of three clinical books of SCM case studies and the top expert of the body measuring system for diagnosing Sasang constitutions in Korea. Without his help in reviewing the original Korean text, editing this book would have been impossible.

I believe this publication will open the minds and hearts of those who wish to benefit from a holistic philosophy toward better health and longevity. Better health through the advancement of Sasang Constitutional Medicine will greatly improve the lives of others living in both Eastern and Western civilization.

Floyd E. Sandoval
Seoul, South Korea
October 2004

Contents

Chapter 3. Daily Health Maintenance Using Sasang Constitutional Theory

Part II. Understanding Sasang Constitutional Medicine

Chapter 4. Understanding Sasang Constitutional Medicine

Chapter 5. Teachings on Health Cultivation by Dr. Lee Je-ma

Part I

Achieving Health through Knowledge of Your Constitution

Chapter 1
Achieving Health through Knowledge of Your Constitution

Sasang medicine is a constitutional medicine. Each and every person is one of four constitutions; *Soeumin, Tae-eumin, Soyangin* or *Taeyangin.* What are the benefits of knowing your constitution? This question will be answered in the first chapter, "Achieving Health through Knowledge of Your Constitution." When differentiating constitutions, the shape of the physical body and the person's mental tendencies are the two important attributes to consider. Because each constitution has different strengths and weaknesses, appropriate healing foods and tonics will differ among constitutions, as will reactions to disease and proper treatment methods. The way that each constitution specifically reacts to healing foods and tonics, disease and various treatments must be understood in order to successfully practice constitutional medicine.

Let us now begin our discussion with the following six themes:

1. Yang Kuei-fei and Cleopatra
2. It's Your Fault
3. The Story of Pork and Chicken
4. The Story of Ginseng & Deer Horn
5. Those with Upper Body Problems and Those with Lower Body Problems
6. Will a Physically Weak Person Have Longevity?

1. Yang Kuei-fei and Cleopatra

What subjects do modern women look to read about in magazines? Politics, scandal, news, gossip, fashion, art and entertainment are all areas of common interest. However, in today's culture, it seems that reading about new techniques for maintaining youth and beauty is of particular appeal. There is a constant search for that miracle wrinkle cream, weight loss product or other external solution to preserve the look of youth and beauty.

The desire to maintain beauty can be insatiable. This universal desire has led to the creation of an enormous cosmetics industry, devoted to providing superficial improvements to women's appearance. Highly advanced science and technology is used to help women achieve unnatural, cosmetic beauty. Similarly, science and technology is also used to assist weight loss, either through diets or medical procedures.

For hundreds of years, western and eastern cultures have had different standards of feminine beauty. Western society favors a well-proportioned figure, whereas easterners love the oval-shaped outline of the face. Simply stated, westerners focus on the outline of the body or the trunk, while easterners focus on the face and its feature.

In the past, eastern custom forbade people to look at the globalization, western-style clothes that emphasize a woman's figure have become commonplace in the east, part of the effect of which has been to alter previous eastern conceptions of female beauty. Using today's standards, neither traditional Asian beauty Yang Kuei-fei[1] (719-756 AD) nor Chun-hyang[2] would be considered a first-class beauty. No matter how hard Yang Kuei-fei or Chun-hyang exercised or kept a strict dietary regimen, there is no guarantee that they would win the Miss Korea beauty pageant. This is because a person's appearance and bodily shape are prenatally determined and will not change significantly regardless of postnatal efforts.

People have one head, one trunk, two arms and two legs. So why is it that some women have an hourglass figure, while

---

1) During the time of the Tang Dynasty, 18th son of King Xuan Zong was married to a beautiful Chinese performer called Yang Kuei-fei. Her beauty was so well known that King Xuan Zong wanted her to perform for him. At his request, she danced and sang songs the king had written himself. King Xuan Zong was so charmed by her beauty and seductive dance that he fell deeply in love and began to treat her as the Empress. This obsession eventually led to his destruction; the king neglected his duties and responsibilities to his kingdom, and immediately became the target of an assassination plot by his political enemies. A civil war broke out in the kingdom (the war of An Lui Shan) in 755AD. Finally, his military chiefs ordered Yang Kuei-fei to be hanged in 756AD.

2) Pansori Chun-hyang (a Korean opera) tells the story of Chun-hyang, a fictional character known to be the most beautiful woman in Korea. Here is her story:

Chun-hyang's beauty was well known throughout the land. One day she met a young man who promised to marry her after he completed his government examination to be an agent of the king. Having this young man's promise, Chun-hyang was determined to reject all other offers of marriage and remain single waiting for his return. Soon after his departure, an evil government tax collector ordered her to serve him as his personal assistant. His intentions were immoral and she rejected his demands. Infuriated by her repeated rejections, he had her jailed and made her wear a large wooden yoke around her neck. She was given three days to comply with his wishes or she would be put to death. Chun-hyang's devotion was so strong that she refused to comply with the wishes of the evil man even though she was facing certain death. At the very moment the government tax collector was going to have Chun-hyang flogged to death, her fiancée returned as the secret royal inspector and agent of the king. With his new authority he ordered the wicked tax collector be arrested and jailed for the abusive illegal demand she placed on Chun-hyang. After being liberated she was able to marry her true love and live happily ever after.

others are stout and plump? Why is it that some men can take pride in their strong physique and square shoulders, while others have thin physique with sloping shoulders?

The answer is that a body type is determined by the relative strengths and weaknesses of certain internal organs. Each person is born with a specific constitution that arises from innate differences in the strengths of those organs. Sasang Constitutional Medicine (SCM) explains that one's body is composed of four different regions: the Upper Burner, Upper-Middle Burner, Lower-Middle Burner, and Lower Burner. The organs contained within these regions are the Lungs, Spleen, Liver and Kidneys, respectively. People with sufficient Lung energy have thick necks and square-shoulders, displaying manly physiques. However, they are lacking in Liver energy so they appear weak when standing, as their bodies are weaker below the waist. In contrast, people with strong Kidney energy have wide hips and strong legs, but they have narrow shoulders. Their overall body shape is the most feminine of the four constitutions.

In general, *yang* constitutions (*Soyangin* and *Taeyangin*) have well-developed upper bodies with weak lower bodies, while *yin* constitutions (*Soeumin* and *Tae-eumin*) have stronger lower bodies and weaker upper bodies. A woman with a slim waist, wide hips, and neat appearance would likely be *Soeumin.* While *Soeumin* women generally have the most feminine or shapely figure, *Soeumin* men are generally neat in their appearance.

Frequently, we see beautiful women dressed in modern clothing wearing high heels to accentuate their physical beauty. Sometimes we see ladies who look just as good wearing casual clothing with flat bottom shoes. Some women can wear almost anything and look great, while other women who wear the same thing might not look as good because of their particular constitution. Nature, however, distributes strengths and weaknesses equally to all people. Therefore a person does not need to be disappointed that a certain outfit does not fit her well.

It seems that young women in today's society are overly

concerned with their physical appearances. Should it matter if some girls are little clumsy and overweight? Should they not be thankful for their health? It is quite sad to see some ladies overly indulging in extravagant beauty ointments and cosmetics for idle vanity, while many are dying of accidents and diseases. Excessive dietary measures may temporarily give a person some happiness in terms of weight loss, but it is not known whether or not this extreme dieting may shorten a person's life by tens of years.

True beauty with its idiosyncrasies of one's natural personality and character can only arise from good health. People will never tire of gazing at this natural beauty no matter how long they look. But if a woman loses too much weight, or undergoes plastic surgery, or receives laser treatments or any other cosmetic treatments, would she not damage her health or natural bone structure using methods that are not appropriate for her physical frame?

This is also true for men. Not everyone can have the physique of Michelangelo's David sculpture. *Soeumin* men do not need to be ashamed of their body shape, which is most likely slim and small in stature. There are many women who love this shape and the tidy appearance of *Soeumin* men so they will have no trouble finding a good spouse. Tall men really have no advantage in life except that they can reach things in high places more easily. Thick, muscular men do not derive any additional enjoyment from life other than the excitement they may gain from being able to overflow the water in the bathtub when they submerge themselves.

By maintaining the rules of health that correspond to each body type, it is possible to make one's body beautiful naturally. Not only will your body be healthy but your mind will also be clear so that your whole being will become more attractive. Let us live our lives according to our own characteristics! Or better yet, let us live our lives according to our constitutions! Isn't this the key to true beauty?

The physical shape and features of the body vary with the constitution.

This is the first proposition we have to bear in mind.

2. It's Your Fault

When observing people individually, we see that some may shine when working alone but get lost when working in a group environment. Others stand out prominently working within a group but have difficulty working alone. People display a wide variety of living styles. There are also many differences in patterns of social and business activities. These all depend upon individual psychological differences. According to SCM, personalities and mental dispositions vary across each constitutional type. Some people prefer solitude and find social interactions difficult, while others relish social activities and are incapable of maintaining their own personal affairs.

Yang types, like *Soyangins* and *Taeyangins*, are progressive and have the ability to stand out in a crowd. Their vice is that they tend to be overly aggressive. When they fail at any endeavor it is generally due to a lack of precision and deliberation. In addition, *yang* types have a difficult time handling their domestic affairs because their focus is primarily on external matters. In contrast, *Tae-eumins* and *Soeumins* make their personal affairs a top priority. Social relationships are secondary. They try to solve difficult problems on their own and take full responsibility for their actions. Their vice is that they do not like outside intervention in their affairs, so they suffer alone even when a problem could easily be solved with a little advice or help from others.

In a group environment, *Taeyangins* and *Soyangins* believe that the duty of each member of the group will unfold if one person takes the initiative as the group leader. But *Tae-eumins* and *Soeumins* believe that if each member of the group does his or her part, the goal of the group will be pursued and obtained automatically. Obviously the most desirable group dynamic is a harmonious environment shared by all four constitutions.

The strength and efficiency of an organization depend upon the strengths of different people in their designated positions. If disharmony exists between various members who have different inclinations, then there will be discord and perhaps a quarrel or two.

It is well known that the majority of salaried workers are under a great deal of stress and the majority of people who abruptly quit their jobs do so because of troubled relations with coworkers. Troubled relationships with either coworkers or superiors are much more common than issues with company policies or procedures.

The two basic thought patterns that create problems in human relations are "fault finding in others" and "envy or jealousy (the grass is always greener on the other side)." These two traits are commonly seen in the *Taeyangin* and *Soeumin* types.

Taeyangins are progressive. They set plans and work whole-heartedly to achieve them. Too often, however, they do not achieve their goals because they lack precision. They find fault in others and project their own failures onto anyone who has not followed their exact instructions. The members of a department headed by a *Taeyangin* will often find themselves out at bars together after work, either to unite when they are planning and pursuing a goal or to complain about their supervisor when they fail.

Soeumins are gentle and passive. However, there are many times that they feel jealous of the successes of others and they tend to hold grudges for a long time if they are offended. Though they are very often displeased with other people's planning abilities, they refuse to take the lead. In carrying out plans, they usually over-analyze things, which allow others to take the initiative. It is these characteristics that will lead a *Soeumin*, in an extreme situation, to become jealous of the success of others and try to find fault with the work of others. In a department headed by a supervisor with these characteristics, intelligent plans made by subordinates are likely to be ignored for no apparent reason. In addition, highly intelligent employees can bring about jealousy in their supervisor, which makes it difficult to achieve harmony in the workplace.

These negative traits may draw an overly pessimistic picture of the *Soeumins*. However, if the head of a department is a *Soeumin*, although they may be reluctant to start a new project, once it is started the *Soeumin* will plan out the details meticulously and will make few mistakes. In a department with *Taeyangin* at the helm, the department will be able to carry out plans in a dynamic fashion as long as there is ample support from conscientious employees.

According to the principles of SCM, constitutional differences account for variations in not only body shape and countenance, but also in mental dispositions. In general, *Taeyangins* are aggressive and self-righteous, *Soyangins* are strong and sharp, *Tae-eumins* are slow and taciturn, and *Soeumins* are gentle and scrupulous.

It is important to keep in mind that inherent in each constitution are differences in characteristics, personalities and talents. The key to better social relationships is to successfully maintain relationships with people whose constitutions differ from your own. This way you can make use of their strengths in order to counter your own temperamental weaknesses.

SCM is not only reliable in treating physical disorders but also offers wisdom with which we can improve our lives because it urges us to take precautions against certain harmful elements. It enables us to cultivate our inherent strengths, and modify our inherent weaknesses according to individual constitutions.

Mental dispositions vary according to the different constitutions.

This is the second proposition we have to remember.

3. The Story of Pork and Chicken

Many people in Korea believe that eating pork or chicken can cause a stroke. In fact, some people have stopped eating pork and chicken altogether. Others know not to take herbal prescriptions with pork and chicken. It does not seem right to condemn pork and chicken outright particularly if you evaluate these two foods from the perspective of western nutritional science, which claims that pork and chicken have plenty of essential amino and fatty acids.

Interestingly, although pork and chicken are frowned upon, beef is welcomed. In Korea, serving beef to guests is a display of generosity because beef is more expensive than pork or chicken. However, simply being more expensive does not imply that the food is healthier.

From the viewpoint of SCM, there's no rationale for the belief that beef is better than pork or chicken. The effect that each food has on the body differs according to the constitution of an individual. For example, for *Soeumins*, chicken and lamb are healthier than pork or beef.

Though *Soeumins* do better avoiding pork, a little pork will do them no harm. If eating a small amount of pork had a great effect, the pork would be reacting like medicine rather than like a food. Traditionally, foods and medicines are said to have come from the same source but differ greatly in potency. Because food is much less potent than medicine, there will not be a great reaction with a small quantity.

Food supplies our bodies with dynamic energy and fundamental elements so it is important that our diets are diverse. By eating a variety of foods, the unbalanced nature of one food will be balanced by other foods, thus preventing problems for the constitution. In SCM, foods are selected for each constitution in order to treat diseases and as a precaution for those who maintain a diet that is inappropriate for their constitution.

SCM does not consider one type of meat superior to any other. Each constitution has its own peculiarities. Such peculiarities need to be understood, and people need to examine their diets and make appropriate corrections in order to maintain balance. Although food is not as strong as medicine, it is eaten continuously, unlike medicine, which is usually prescribed on a short-term basis. Thus, in the long run, food might have a stronger effect than medicine, as it accumulates in the body.

Taeyangins should avoid foods that are spicy, warm or greasy, as they are not appropriate for their body type. They will be better off with bland and cool foods. *Soyangins* should avoid warm and stimulating foods. They would do better with cold and raw foods. *Tae-eumins* should stay away from greasy and stimulating foods and eat foods that are high in protein. *Soeumins* should not eat cold and greasy foods; rather they should try to eat warm and slightly stimulating foods.

Foods need to be eaten according to differing constitutions.

This is the third principle to remember.

4. The Story of Ginseng & Deer Horn

Ginseng is a tonic herb that is considered a superior herb according to the book, *Shen Nung's Herbal* (*Shennung bencao jing*). Ginseng that is not processed is called "raw ginseng," while ginseng that is dried under the sun is called "white ginseng." "Red ginseng" is steamed in a specific way and dried. The property of ginseng is slightly warm and non-toxic, and it has a slightly bitter taste. It is difficult to enumerate all of its effects because of its extensive use.

Of all herbs, the functions and ingredients of ginseng are currently the most thoroughly researched due to its wide range of effects. This research has been conducted using modern technology and modern instruments. As a result, ginseng's effectiveness has been scientifically validated. Because of the research, western science has answered some of the questions about the efficacy of ginseng. It is questionable, however, if and how this research has affected the eastern medical view of ginseng's capabilities.

The "deer horn (*lu rong*)" is the newly grown horn of a deer that is gathered, processed and dried. If the horn is not cut but is left to grow, it will ossify from calcium deposits. This ossified horn is also an herb and is called *lu jiao* (cornu cervi). The horn that naturally falls off one year later is called *lo jiao*. The uses of all three herbs are similar, but their therapeutic effects and prices vary greatly. When deer horn is cooked for a long time and made into glue, it is called *lu jiao jiao* (gelatinum cornu cervi). The dregs left over after boiling the deer antler glue is called *lu jiao shuang* (cornu cervi degelatinatium).

Deer horn is warm, and has a sweet and slightly salty or sour taste. Together with ginseng, deer horn is known to be an excellent therapeutic tonic. The only drawback to deer horn is that it is expensive. In Korea, deer horn is expensive, not because of its function, but because of the incredibly high demand.

Those who have used tonics such as ginseng and deer horn have their own opinions as to their effectiveness. There are a lot of people who praise ginseng and use it routinely. Ginseng can be taken on a daily basis, and in different forms. Some people mix ginseng powder in homemade honey, while others boil it with jujubes and drink it as a tea. Still others take it in a convenient pill form.

Despite the popularity and validity of ginseng, there are people who get angry whenever they hear the praises of ginseng because when they use the herb they develop skin rashes and their bodies feel heavy or their symptoms worsen.

There are also conflicting opinions about the effectiveness of deer horn as with ginseng. Some people believe that deer horn is the best herb to promote longevity. Others say that it is simply expensive and does not have any real benefits. Some people even believe that there are severe side effects from ingesting deer horn, such as mental retardation in children, which is untrue.

All of these statements are over-generalizations. Ginseng and deer horn are unparalleled tonics but their effects are due to their unique functions. They do not affect every person in the same way. They can exhibit completely different effects depending on an individual's constitution or symptoms.

The previously mentioned person who got skin rashes and a fever after taking ginseng is probably *Soyangin*. Ginseng is not appropriate for *Soyangins* who constitutionally have heat in the Spleen and Stomach. When using herbal formulas for these people, ginseng can be taken out or it can be substituted with sea cucumber, otherwise known as sea ginseng. Ginseng is most appropriate for *Soeumin*. It is used in almost every prescription for *Soeumin*.

Since the *Tae-eumin* constitution has a weak Lung function, it is best to use herbs that strengthen the Lung. Deer horn or bear gallbladder, two of the most expensive herbs in Eastern medicine, are good for the weak Lung function in *Tae-eumins*. It is not necessary, however, to over-emphasize either deer horn or bear gallbladder since their price alone does not guarantee their effectiveness. Regardless of the cost, it is the relationship that an herbal remedy has with your constitution that will give you the desired results.

Because herbal tonics are expensive, people would attempt to find less expensive alternatives if they thought that they would have the same effect. If bear gallbladder is too pricey, perhaps pig gallbladder can be substituted for a lesser price. Unfortunately, the constitutionally specific reaction may not be achieved. Some people choose to purchase expensive herbal prescription that costs up to $400 or $500 as a gift, thinking that if it costs more it must work better. It is important to remember that good health cannot be bought. Without the knowledge of an individual's constitution, signs and symptoms, buying expensive tonic herbs will likely have very little effect on a person's health.

This is not limited to tonic herbs. The eastern herbal pharmacy contains both warm and cold herbs. If a particular herb is not suitable for an individual constitution, it cannot be used even if the herb is indicated for the symptoms.

Some tonic herbs can be toxic if they do not match the constitution.

This is the fourth principle to remember.

5. Those with Upper Body Problems and Those with Lower Body Problems

If you do not enjoy your food and drink, half of your life will be boring. If you have no appetite, suffer from abdominal bloating, pain in the epigastrium, or nausea, then you will most likely be depressed and irritable. These problems occur for some people on a daily basis for their entire lives.

Some people have digestive problems while others have elimination problems. Some people go to bed at night worrying whether or not they will have a bowel movement the next day and continue to worry about it after they wake up. This may sound strange, but no one can understand the problems these people have without having experienced the same symptoms.

Western medicine has been unsuccessful in finding and treating the root causes of stomach problems and constipation. In most cases, digestive enzymes and antacids are prescribed. Laxatives give only temporary symptomatic relief. For these reasons, the majority of people who suffer these conditions feel that they are destined to endure their problems for the rest of their lives.

Unlike western medicine, Eastern medicine emphasizes the importance of treating stomach disorders and constipation and it has devised a means to treat the root causes of these disorders. In Eastern medicine, the names given to the diseases such as "gastritis," "gastric ulcers," and "gastroptosis" are not very significant. It focuses instead upon generating treatment methods that address the root causes of the stomach and intestinal weaknesses.

Knowing how internal organs function can lead to a better understanding of how to successfully treat an ailment. For example, if the stomach disorder is caused by phlegm and dampness that arises from a weakness in the absorbing function of the stomach created by an internal coldness, a formula such as *Erchen tang* (Two Aged Peel Decoction) is prescribed. For gastroptosis, which is due to Stomach *qi* deficiency, formulas such as *Renshenyangwei tang* (Nourish the Stomach with Ginseng Decoction) or *Buzhongyiqi tang* (Tonify the Middle and Augment the *qi* Decoction) can be prescribed to restore balance. If there is little appetite and gastritis, *Pingwei san* (Harmonize the Stomach Powder) is used first followed by *Shenzhujianpi tang* (Rebuild the Spleen with Ginseng and Atractylodes Decoction).

In Eastern medicine, strong purgatives are used cautiously for constipation. There are generally two major causes of constipation. One is heat in the Stomach Channel, and the other is *qi* deficiency in the Large Intestine due to blood stagnation. On occasion herbal prescriptions are not as effective as they should be. More than likely the reason is a misdiagnosis of the constitution. *Soeumin* is susceptible to stomach problems, but if you use a *Soeumin* prescription for another constitution, it simply won't work.

From the perspective of SCM, *Soeumins* display a tendency to digestive problems in the upper GI, while *Tae-eumins* display a tendency towards problems in the lower GI and frequently suffer from constipation. If *Soeumins* have constipation it simply means that they have eaten food that is not appropriate for their constitution. *Tae-eumins* enjoy eating and drinking because they do not suffer from digestive problems. However, they are commonly faced with sweating and elimination problems. If these problems persist they can be a cause of illness.

Each constitution must be wary of certain diseases. In addition, even though the ailments may be the same, such as stomach disease and constipation, the symptoms that arise from these ailments will not manifest in the same way nor will they affect each constitution in the same way. Ailments need to be treated according to body type in order to be effectively and fundamentally treated. So, as you can see, one ailment can have different treatments according to the constitutional makeup of a particular person.

Traditionally it is said that a single disease can have ten thousand different remedies. This variety is not solely a product of a variation of symptoms. It is fundamentally due to constitutional differences, which are responsible for the diversity of causes and progressions of a disease.

The treatment method of SCM varies greatly from the syndrome differentiating method of TCM (Syndrome Medicine). While SCM concentrates on finding the root cause of the problem and treats it accordingly, Syndrome Medicine often treats deficiencies and excesses using tonifying and sedating techniques. Specially, SCM distinguishes herbs for each constitution. If an herb is not proper for a certain constitution, it will not be used in a formula even though the symptom may be indicated.

Each constitution has its own category of diseases and corresponding treatment principles.

This is the fifth principle to remember.

6. Will a Physically Weak Person Have Longevity?

What is the standard for a healthy life? If you consider the length of life as a standard of health, will a physically weak person have longevity?

There once was a man who had a chronic cough, yet he lived more than 90 years. Can you believe that a man with a weak constitution, who catches a cold almost every month, and eats only small amount of food, could live to be more than 70 or 80 years of age? Have you ever heard the adage, "He who has asthma lives long."?

Believe it or not, there is a story of famous doctor Bian

Xue (*circa* 407-310 BC) whose father was very old and suffered greatly from chronic asthma. Bian Xue's disciples could not understand why Bian Xue, the most famous doctor of his time, could not heal his own father's asthma. Therefore, his disciples, thinking they knew the proper treatment and wanting to show off their skills, treated Bian Xue's father's symptoms with ease. When Bian Xue discovered what had happened, he said, "Oh, my goodness, my father's life is now over!" As he predicted, his father died one month later.

There is an old saying that makes the claim that health and longevity do not depend on the strength of an individual. People with weak constitutions tend to take better care of their health because they are always very conscious about their own health problems. Even though they have not learned SCM, they are very sensitive to harmful factors because they understand the weakness of their condition. These people have no difficulty in attaining longevity, even though they may look weak or frequently fall ill. In contrast, people who are used to being in good health suffer unexpected health crisis around middle age. Even though they may be strong physically and have an excellent digestive system, if they are overconfident about their health and continue an immoderate lifestyle without putting forth effort to maintain good health, they will not be able to defend themselves against an unexpected ailment. Even the strongest steel can be crushed once its weakness is discovered, despite its indestructible appearance.

It is important to pay special attention to healthy living habits, especially when recovering from an illness. It can take an entire lifetime to attain good health, but it only takes a moment of carelessness to destroy it. Elderly people quickly interrupt the statement "I have good health. I've never even caught a cold" with a solemn look.

According to the SCM tradition, *Soeumins* appear to be weak. But *Soeumins* are scrupulous, so they are very cautious in their actions, thereby preventing disasters. In light of this, any one constitution does not equate good health. A constitution is determined at birth; however, each individual is responsible for regulating his or her own body's constitutional needs.

In general, every constitution has its own merits and demerits. There is not one particular constitution that remains entirely free of disease and enjoys longevity. If every person were to be educated about their own constitution, they would be able to rid themselves of its weaknesses and promote its strengths, thereby enjoying freedom from disease and achieving longevity.

The next chapter will discuss the practical method of identifying Sasang constitutions.

Chapter 2
Methods of Differentiating Sasang Constitutions

The Sasang constitutional theory of Dr. Lee Je-ma is arguably the most comprehensive systematized constitutional theory in the world. Prior to the development of Sasang theory the concept of constitution was obscure in both the East and the West. Consequently, much of constitutional theory was not practically applied to treat diseases.

Dr. Lee Je-ma identified four Sasang constitutions, *Taeyangin, Tae-eumin*, *Soyangin*, and *Soeumin*. He explained the physiological and pathological characteristics of each, and described appropriate, corresponding pharmacological treatments. So what distinguishes the four Sasang constitutions?

This chapter suggests various methods for identifying each of the constitutions. After reviewing this chapter, you should be able to recognize your own constitution. If you cannot, it is recommended that you read Chapter 4 and then reread this chapter to gain further clarification on how to recognize and comprehend your constitution.

I. The Three Indexes of Distinguishing Constitutions

In SCM the three most important factors in differentiating constitutions are external appearance, mental characteristics and disease symptoms. External appearance is viewed in terms of the shape of the body and its countenance. Each constitution has its own particular body shape caused by the differences in the size and development of the internal organs, so in many instances observing the shape of the body reveals the constitution. The body will change over the course of a lifetime due to factors that influence physical growth such as nutrition and disease.

In addition, exercise and physical habits can also influence the shape of the body. Nevertheless, the basic body shape remains unchanged. The ideas of body shape discussed in this chapter will give generalities about each constitutional type. However, because there are exceptions, it is not enough to only look at the shape of the body when identifying constitutions. One must also examine a person's mental characteristics and disease symptoms.

Identifying constitutions by examining mental characteristics includes observing a person's temperament, talents, constant state of mind (an innate state of mind maintained by a person of a given constitution throughout his or her lifetime — see the next section), personality, mental desire, etc. Each constitution has its own particular characteristics; therefore observing mental characteristics plays a role in constitutional differentiation. It is, however, difficult to bc objective when trying to identify one's own constitution. Although one might subjectively consider oneself to be an introvert, in reality it can be very difficult to objectively measure that characteristic. Also, there are some people who do not express their mental characteristics outwardly. In such cases, placing them in an unfamiliar situation and observing their reactions can provide a clue in determining their true mental disposition.

Just as normal, healthy physiological conditions vary across each constitution, so do disease signs and symptoms. These disease manifestations can therefore be used to identify a particular constitution. The disease symptoms are first divided into mild and severe, but this division is not sufficient. Each constitution has a typical disease syndrome, but some constitutions show symptoms only when a disease is severe. As previously mentioned, the size and development of the internal organs determine the constitution.

For reference, there was a recent attempt to relate Sasang constitutions to the four blood types (A, B, O and AB). It was hypothesized that there is a relationship between the four constitutions and the four blood types because they are both unchanging constitutional principles and because there are some differences in personality according to blood type. The theory posited that *Taeyangin* relates to AB blood type, *Tae-eumin* to O, *Soeumin* to A, and *Soyangin* to B. Subsequent research showed no correlation between blood types and Sasang constitutions. Even though *Taeyangin* is a rare constitution, there are many people who have AB blood. This alone indicates that the theory is flawed.

Since interest in SCM is steadily increasing, there will be a time when diagnosing one's constitution will be done simply through physiological examination of the DNA.

2. The Characteristics of Physical Appearance Reflecting Each Constitution

According to SCM, there are differences in the development of various regions of the body. Therefore, the particular characteristics of a constitution will manifest in the physical appearance in proportion to the development of the internal organs.

For example, *Taeyangins* who have *yang* body types have well-developed upper bodies (the *yang* region) manifesting as strong chest muscles, while their lower bodies (*yin*) are weak. In contrast, *Soeumins* who have *yin* body types have weaker upper bodies (*yang*) and strong lower body (*yin*) development manifesting as large and well-developed buttocks.

The characteristics of physical appearance in each constitution are as follows:

1) *Taeyangin*

Taeyangins have well-developed upper bodies. The neck region is thick and strong and the head is large. However, the region below the waist tends to be weak. The hips are small and the leg muscles are thin. Thus, in a standing position *Taeyangins* seem unstable. Since the lower body is weak, *Taeyangins* have difficult in walking or standing for a long time. Their facial features are clearly defined and they have thin bodies.

Taeyangin women, who are otherwise healthy, may have difficulty in conceiving. Because they have an innate weakness in the low back and waist, their uterine development may also be weak.

On the whole, this constitution is the most difficult to recognize because it has the lowest percentage (less than 0.1% of the population) of the four constitutions.

2) *Soyangin*

The chest and shoulder regions of the *Soyangin* constitutions are strong and well-developed while the region below the hips is weak. On the whole, since their upper bodies are strong and their lower bodies are slight, *Soyangins*' movements are quick. Since their hip region is weak, they also appear weak in a sitting position.

Some *Soyangins* are small in stature and have a tidy appearance, resembling *Soeumins*. It is therefore difficult at times to reach a conclusion about a constitution based solely on the physical appearance. In this case, mental characteristics and disease symptoms must be carefully observed in order to avoid misdiagnosis. There is a high proportion of *Soyangins* in the population and they are fairly easy to distinguish.

3) *Tae-eumin*

The *Tae-eumin* constitution has a well-developed waist region so their standing posture appears stable and strong. Their neck region, however, appears weak. *Tae-eumins* are normally tall and well built and rarely thin and small. Usually, *Tae-eumins* hold ample flesh and their physical frame is stout (strong and solid). On occasion a *Tae-eumin* may be thin, but nevertheless, his or her frame will be stout.

Even though the *Tae-eumins* manifest clear traits, there are cases in which it is difficult to ascertain their constitution, and so it is not enough to rely solely on external appearances. In particular, since *Tae-eumins'* outward appearances share traits with those of *Soeumins*, caution is needed when determining their constitutions.

4) *Soeumin*

Soeumins' hips and buttocks are well-developed and their seated posture is stable, but their chest and shoulder regions appear weak and underdeveloped. *Soeumins* are usually short in stature but at times tall *Soeumins* can be found. Their lower bodies are more balanced and developed than their upper bodies. Many *Soeumins* tend to walk with their bodies bent forward. Although their lower bodies are generally more developed than their upper bodies, on the whole, they have small frames and are thin and weak.

Since female *Soeumins*, in contrast to female *Taeyangins*, have large hips and a well-developed uterus, they can get pregnant easily and have few problems carrying a child full term.

3. The Mental Characteristics Reflecting Each Constitution

The most important feature of SCM is that it is a mind-body medicine that views the mind and the body as one. Instead of considering the mind and body separately, SCM stresses the intimate relationship of the mind to the physical characteristics. In the same way that physical shape varies according to one's constitution, so do mental characteristics.

Psychological differences appear in several forms. In SCM, these differences include skills and talents (ability, temperament, virtues, etc.), constant state of minds, mental desires and so forth. These psychological differences bring about differences in social activities such as aptitudes, personal and social relationships, the way work is handled, etc. Other factors that need to be taken into account are education, environment and mental cultivation. These factors can alter a person's constant state of mind and other mental characteristics.

1) *Taeyangin*

(1) Skills and Talents

Taeyangins have a great ability to communicate when socializing with others and are resolute in nature. They are very capable in social relationships not because they are gentle and affectionate like *Soeumins*, but because they approach social relationships without reserve or hesitation and they have extremely positive attitudes. (This is called having talent for "social acquaintances.")

(2) Constant State of Mind

Taeyangins have an urgent mind, which indicates a quick temper. They have to control their hot temper in order to regulate the Liver blood. The times when *Taeyangins* are living and working harmoniously are when they are exercising self-control and are able to stay calm. If they are overstrained and pushed to their limits, then their urgent mind appears to impede their work and damage their health.

(3) Personality

Taeyangins are always attempting to rush forward without looking back and they exhibit masculine characteristics rather than feminine ones. What this implies is that they are very courageous and positive.

(4) Mental Desires

Taeyangins have a self-indulgent mind. When there is a greater inclination to exhibit masculine rather than feminine traits, the mind becomes self-indulgent. *Taeyangins* are always rushing forward without reflection, are rash without introspection, and strong without tenderness or sensitivity. When these mental states are in the extreme, the mind becomes self-indulgent, causing them to act in any way that pleases them. If this state is maintained, no one will want to give them advice.

On a positive note, *Taeyangins* are the type of leaders that act with resoluteness. This, however, predisposes them to act as dictators. Their masculine traits have the merit of positive and progressive thinking as well as decisiveness. But they also have vices such as self-righteousness and a lack of planning or precision. They act without hesitation or regret. *Taeyangins* are very good at communicating with others regardless of the relationship. When *Taeyangins* have problems with a plan they are pursuing, however, they easily become angered at others.

2) *Soyangin*

(1) Skills and Talents

Soyangins' strengths lie in being strong and quick. They are skilled in management and carrying forward with plans (This is called having talent for appointing roles[3].”). As members of a *yang* constitution, *Soyangins* exhibit strength and a positive attitude so that they have no trouble beginning new projects.

Soyangins do not hesitate nor do they calculate or worry over details. Instead they launch into new projects readily. Their active demeanor and quick movements make them look highly spirited, not clumsy or awkward.

(2) Constant State of Mind

Soyangins constantly carry anxiety within them. They easily progress with any type of work, but have trouble completing the work once it is started. They have the habit of continuously beginning new projects and leaving them unfinished. They can encounter frequent problems from so many simultaneous ventures, which is why they are so anxious over what may go wrong. When this situation occurs frequently and they have to face serious problems that cause psychological trauma, their anxiety becomes increasingly severe. If they cannot suppress this anxiety so that it develops into a state of fear, it will lead to forgetfulness. This indicates that the condition is serious.

(3) Personality

Soyangins are always starting projects without organizing or completing them. They tend to focus on external affairs and neglect domestic matters. Since their work is usually not completed and not cared for, family members or coworkers have a hard time dealing with them. In many situations, a *Soyangin* will begin a project but someone else will have to finish it.

Soyangins like to receive praise and compliments and strive towards fame. They do not find a great deal of satisfaction in working earnestly on domestic affairs. Although they find great pleasure in helping others, they are less pleased with domestic work.

---

3) the induction, organization and management of work.

(4) Mental Desires

The *Soyangins'* disposition tends to have partiality. When *Soyangins* try to accomplish outside affairs without regulating their inner or domestic affairs, they are carried away by their personal emotions. *Soyangins* do not exercise moderation or prioritize their work. They do not clearly differentiate between what is necessary or unnecessary, important or unimportant, private or public, and instead they simply work according to their moods or emotions. When this occurs, they act and behave according to their moods and feelings. Because of this, others think that they have no principles (disorganized) and find that they are less dependable to work with.

Soyangins are both positive and quick, and so are good at starting and managing affairs. They are also very active and passionate, honest and frank, and have a strong chivalrous and altruistic spirit. Though they may be hasty and carefree, they are very compassionate and are not really genuinely interested in profit and loss. Their vice, however, is their hastiness and inattentiveness toward themselves and their family members because they are always focused on outside matters. They are also easily bored and frequently give up on projects that they have begun. That is, they lack perseverance or persistence.

3) *Tae-eumin*

(1) Skills and Talents

Tae-eumins are persistent and calm. No matter what task they attempt, once the work is initiated they are able to finish it. *Tae-eumins* have a talent for adjusting themselves to whatever environment they are in and are capable administrators.(This is called having talent for adjusting to their own environment.). Due to their persistence, *Tae-eumins* do not give up easily even though they may encounter some difficulties. They can sit still for a long time and complete work that needs to be done. If a certain project is not finished, they feel very uncomfortable.

(2) Constant State of Mind

Tae-eumins always carry fear (caution) within them. When they are calm, their social and family lives as well as their work are stable so that they earn trust from others. However, if *Tae-eumins* become overly cautious, they become fearful of any work, even before they attempt it, and so they accomplish nothing. As this fear is a constant hindrance for *Tae-eumins*, they dislike any type of change. They immerse themselves in their present state or situation. When the fear becomes greater, serious disease such as palpitations can occur.

(3) Personality

Tae-eumins like to stay calm and dislike moving. They dislike change and are conservative. They try only to accomplish what they can within their own given boundaries and do not want to contend in the outside world. They set their own boundaries in their families and their work, and are not interested in other people's work. It is rare that a *Tae-eumin* would put any effort into acquiring a vain, empty reputation as a *Soyangin* might do.

(4) Mental Desires

Tae-eumins have a greedy nature. If they have an excessive need to maintain their own boundaries, greed may hinder their lives. Although accomplishing their goals and maintaining their possessions can be beneficial, if they become overly attached to their possessions, they will become greedy.

Tae-eumins have an imposing countenance and demeanor and strong conversational skills. They look calm, are impartial and can efficiently organize all types of work. Because *Tae-eumins* are honest and exercise caution, they are trustworthy. *Tae-eumins* are conservative and courteous. They are able to achieve success in their business due to persistent efforts and great patience.

Tae-eumins give priority to their family and not to outside affairs. Although their outer appearance seems gentle, there is a lot of doubt and greed inside. They dislike activity and chatting, and prefer recreational activities to sports. Their vices include excessive fear (overly cautious), dullness, and indolence.

Historically, there have been many heroes and patriots who belonged to the *Tae-eumin* constitution. However, there have also been many *Tae-eumins* of precarious character that succumb to weak mentality and will, narrow-mindedness, indolence, and dullness.

4) *Soeumin*

(1) Skills and Talents

Soeumins have the virtue of being courteous and calm. They are capable organizers of people because they are prudent and kind (This is called having talent for "clanships."). They are also very meticulous planners regardless of the undertaking. *Soeumins* interact well with others because they are sensitive to the needs of others.

(2) Constant State of Mind

Soeumins are constantly nervous. From another perspective, their prudent personality implies that they are timid or fainthearted. Thus, *Soeumins* easily feel anxious and nervous about even minute problems. This nervousness is not only a vice of the *Soeumin* mind; it can also negatively affect their health. Since they worry about every little trifle, *Soeumins* have problems with digestion and often feel a stifling sensation in the chest. When their nervousness is abated, the Spleen *qi* will become vitalized and the *Soeumin* will become healthy.

(3) Personality

Soeumins generally prefer staying home to going out. That is, *Soeumins* are introverted. They tend to exhibit more feminine than masculine characteristics. This implies that they are pessimistic and lack the drive to start things. Nevertheless, they are very meticulous and calm. Though they can get temporarily wrapped up in an emotion, *Soeumins* are the type who act rationally and do not let emotions override them.

(4) Mental Desires

Soeumins tend towards indolence. When there is too much introversion and passiveness, it can easily lead to indolence. Even in a situation where *Soeumins* may achieve great success, they will typically end up with minimal results due to their passive nature. When placed in a difficult situation, *Soeumins* become more passive to avoid even a small adventure, and thus remain endlessly idle. Without risk taking, nothing is accomplished. This idle mind is the mental desire of *Soeumins*.

Soeumins' appearance, mode of speech, and demeanor are natural, graceful, and skillful. They are also docile, calm and social. They make wise decisions and are meticulous and methodical.

However, *Soeumins* are introverted and shy, so they keep most of their opinions to themselves. They have very little drive to accomplish things because of their feminine and passive nature, but their individualism and selfishness are strong. *Soeumins*, therefore, do not like to be bothered by others and tend to count every profit and loss. Also, because they exhibit a great deal of jealousy and envy, they tend to hold on to hurt feelings for a long time.

5) Conclusion

According to the SCM definition of the nature of the mind, if a person's mental nature is clearly manifested, then constitutional differentiation will be easier. There are many individual differences, however, and according to education or life experience, certain characteristics may be more prominent in some people than in others.

The mental nature of each constitution should not be taken

as an absolute. For example, urgency or nervousness does not appear only in *Taeyangins* or *Soeumins*; everyone can feel urgent and nervous at times. These emotions are relative. Everyone has *Four Principles* of the mind (i.e. urgency, anxiety, fear, and nervousness) yet each individual has a predominant characteristic according to his or her constitution.

4. The Disease Syndromes Reflecting Each Constitution

In general, TCM does not associate any one particular disease pattern with any given constitution. In other words, there is no consideration given to the reasons behind why some people are afflicted with certain diseases while others are not. TCM views the human body as an innately harmonized and balanced entity. Diseases arise due to certain factors inside or outside of the body that break that balance. Therefore, Eastern medicine differentiates the unbalanced state into excesses and deficiencies. The treatment principle focuses on restoring balance by eliminating these disruptive factors.

In contrast, SCM views the human body as an inherently incomplete and unbalanced system. Harmony does not arise automatically but can only be obtained by conscious effort. There are imperfections and imbalances not only in the body, but also in the mind. No one is born a sage. It is the basic view of SCM that although one may be born with an unbalanced mind, by cultivating one's mind it is possible to become a sage. Since the body is also not innately balanced, health can only be obtained by controlling one's physical imbalances. Although external factors do, in fact, cause diseases, they do not bring about illness until they affect the internal body. From this perspective, intrinsic factors are considered to be the root cause of diseases.

One symptom can represent either a disease state or a healthy condition depending upon a person's constitution. In addition, each constitution exhibits particular signs of disease as well as particular disease progressions. For example, spontaneous sweating is a healthy sign for *Tae-eumins* but is unhealthy for *Soeumins*. There are also certain diseases that only afflict particular constitutions. In other words, there exist constitutional syndromes. Once these factors are recognized, a natural and effective treatment method can be instituted. Inversely, constitutions can be differentiated through the particular characteristics of constitutional syndromes.

The state of health, aptly called the "healthy state," varies across each constitution. For instance, ease in urination is the healthy state for *Taeyangins*, while sound digestion is the healthy state of *Soeumins*. In the same way, the signs of disease vary according to each constitution. An initial or mild imbalance is known as a "mild disease" and is viewed not only to contrast a healthy state, but also to contrast a "severe disease," which indicates that the disease is either critical or extremely difficult to treat.

In such a way, there are differing states of health and constitutional syndromes, as well as, differing progression of disease in each constitution.

1) *Taeyangin*

(1) Healthy State

Taeyangins are in a healthy state if they urinate a large amount without any difficulty. One way to differentiate a *Taeyangin* is that he or she will have ease in urination when healthy but will have discomfort when not feeling well.

(2) Mild Disease

Taeyangins have a mild disease if they have a great deal of saliva or foam in their mouths. This needs immediate treatment.

(3) Severe Disease

Yul gyuk or dysphagia is the constitutional disease of *Taeyangins*. When this disease worsens, the person will find it difficult to swallow food. Even if he or she is able to swallow the food, it will not descend to the stomach, but instead will be vomited up immediately. At this time, the person can feel slightly cool air flowing up through the esophagus from the stomach area. These symptoms will distinguish a *Taeyangin* and are considered critical symptoms.

Yul gyuk (dysphagia), *ban wyi* (vomiting) and *hae yuk* (lower body weakness) are all important symptoms in differentiating the *Taeyangin* constitution but they do not appear until the situation is serious. Thus *Taeyangins* generally appear to be healthy. *Ban wyi* appears as epigastric bloating and fullness after eating with vomiting afterwards. *Hae yuk* appears as fatigue of the whole body that results in lethargy, weakness of the legs, thinning of the body, and no desire to talk. At times, *yul gyuk* can occur in *Soeumin* elders, so they must not be misdiagnosed as *Taeyangins*.

When a person exhibits the above-mentioned constitutional syndromes and disease progression, the person can be discerned as a *Taeyangin*.

2) *Soyangin*

(1) Healthy State

For *Soyangins*, good bowel movements indicate a healthy state. When the healthy bowel movements turn into constipation as the body becomes ill, the person can be considered to be a *Soyangin*.

Tae-eumins are highly susceptible to constipation. However, it is generally not considered a disease state. In contrast, *Soyangins* are healthy when they have good bowel movements, and unhealthy when they have constipation. Thus, constipation is a clear indication of a disease in *Soyangins*.

(2) Mild Disease

Constipation indicates a mild disease. If a *Soyangin* has constipation, it should be considered as an unhealthy condition and a treatment plan should be devised immediately. Disease progression in the *Soyangin* is quick and so constipation should not be taken lightly.

(3) Severe Disease

When the *Soyangin* has constipation for two or three consecutive days with heat and a stifling sensation in the chest, he or she has a severe disease. In contrast to *Soeumins* who manifest ice-cold abdomens with continuous diarrhea, *Soyangins* will develop a heat sensation in the chest when the constipation continues.

3) *Tae-eumin*

(1) Healthy State

Tae-eumins are in a healthy state if they sweat frequently. If a person sweats easily even though they only move slightly or if they sweat profusely during the wintertime while eating, they are of the *Tae-eumin* constitution. In contrast to *Soeumins* who would feel sick and exhausted after sweating profusely, *Tae-eumins* do not feel even the slightest discomfort; they may actually feel refreshed. A person who sweats in large quantities when there is no disease present has a high probability of being a *Tae-eumin.*

(2) Mild Disease

For the *Tae-eumins,* having firm skin and an inability to sweat indicates a disease state. If there is an absence of sweating, other symptoms will soon follow and the disease will worsen. A person in this state should, therefore, be treated immediately.

(3) Severe Disease

If the Small Intestine (situated in the Lower-Middle Burner) feels blocked as though a fog is clogging up that region, then the disease is considered to be severe.

Usually, profuse sweating is a sign of deficiency or disease. However, in the case of *Tae-eumins,* it is a sign of health. The ideal sweat beads of a *Tae-eumin* are thick and stay on the skin for a long time.

4) *Soeumin*

(1) Healthy State

Soeumins feel healthy when their digestion is good. *Soeumins* generally have weak Spleen *qi,* and so once the Spleen *qi* is revived and digestion is improved, they are in a healthy state. If *Soeumins* have no appetite and develop fullness in the chest after eating, they will feel discomfort.

(2) Mild Disease

Profuse sweating indicates a mild disease. Unlike *Tae-eumins*, spontaneous sweating in *Soeumins* indicates that a disease has already progressed and it must be treated quickly.

(3) Severe Disease

A *Soeumin* with continuous diarrhea and a cold abdomen has a severe disease. This constitution has a weak Spleen and Stomach and so they tend to develop many diseases associated with that weakness. People with chronic digestive problems are usually *Soeumins* and although they may manifest other diseases, these diseases are not of great concern as long as the digestive system is healthy. No matter what the disease, as long as there is no excessive sweating and no problem in drinking water, it is not considered to be a serious disease.

5. Differentiation between *Soeumins* and *Tae-eumins* Must Be Made Carefully

The differentiation between *Soeumin* and *Tae-eumin* is somewhat complicated. If a person is definitely a *yin* type yet distinguishing between *Tae-eumin* and *Soeumin* is difficult, pay attention to the following differences:

- *Soeumins* are in a healthy state when their skin is firm while *Tae-eumins* are not.
- The skin of a *Tae-eumin* is thick while the skin of a *Soeumin* is soft.
- Those who usually have no breathing problems yet sigh at times are *Soeumins*. In contrast, *Tae-eumins* usually do not sigh unless they are exhausted.
- The pulse of *Soeumins* is slightly slow and weak while that of *Tae-eumins* is strong and forceful.
- Those who frequently have symptoms such as palpitations and upward pulling sensation of eyelids, as well as dryness and pain of the eyes can be distinguished as *Tae-eumins*. If there are tremors of the hands and the feet, the person may be *Soeumin*.
- When *Tae-eumins* are afflicted with malaria, they usually want to drink cold water even though they feel chills. This is rare in *Soeumins*, however.
- Spontaneous sweating indicates recovery from an illness in *Tae-eumins*, but worsening of an illness in *Soeumins*.
- *Tae-eumins* in general have large bodies and are seldom small. *Soeumins* generally have small bodies and rarely large bodies in comparison to *Tae-eumins*.
- *Tae-eumins* constantly maintain a fearful mind while *Soeumins* are constantly nervous.
- Appearance, mode of speech, and the demeanors of *Tae-eumins* are dignified, ordered and impartial, while those of *Soeumins* seem natural, light and skillful.

Up to this point the Sasang constitutions have been differentiated into *Taeyangin*, *Tae-eumin, Soyangin* and *Soeumin* types through an explanation of body shapes, the nature of the mind, and disease symptoms. If the characteristics of the Sasang constitutions can be conceived according to these three factors, then you have a clear understanding of the constitutions. Some readers, however, may be unclear about certain parts of the explanation. These readers are advised to envision a more complete picture of the Sasang constitutions.

For example, *Taeyangins* have the strong masculine image of getting furious when their plans fall short of their expectations. *Soyangins* have a different sort of masculine image because they are strong and quick. *Tae-eumins* have a feminine image with voluptuous or plump bodies, while *Soeumins* have a feminine image with small bodies. This method of overlaying different images atop these basic images is effective in order to understand the whole picture.

Correct constitutional differentiation, however, requires a deeper knowledge of SCM. The fourth chapter of this book takes this into consideration and explains its theories in simple terms whenever possible. For those who still have doubts about their constitution, it is recommended that you read Chapter 4 and then return to this chapter. This should enable you to distinguish your own constitution without much difficulty.

<Constitutional Assessment Test>

Questionnaire for the Sasang Classification

A Please read the following questions carefully and mark the answer that best describes you on the answer sheet provided at the end of the book.

1. What is your overall bodily build?
   (a) I have a fairly large size body.
   (b) I have an average size body.
   (c) I have a fairly small size body.
2. What is your body weight relative to your height and overall frame?
   (a) I tend to be overweight.
   (b) I am of an average body weight.
   (c) I am fairly thin.
3. Which of the following statement applies to your body?
   (a) My upper body is stronger and more developed in comparison to my lower body.
   (b) My lower body is stronger and more developed in comparison to my upper body.
   (c) My upper and lower bodies are fairly well proportioned in size and strength.
4. Which of the following most closely matches your bodily shape or build?
   (a) My body resembles an upside down triangle with a well-developed neck and a big head region, but my waist, hips and legs appear weak and underdeveloped.
   (b) My body resembles an upside down triangle with a prominently wide shoulder and chest region tapering down to a fairly narrow waist, hips and buttocks.
   (c) My body resembles that a barrel with a thick waist and protruding abdomen, and a neck region that appears weak and underdeveloped in relation to my overall size.
   (d) My body resembles a ladder with well-developed hips, buttocks and legs but my chest and shoulders appear weak and underdeveloped.
5. How is your overall appearance and physical frame?
   (a) I have thick bones with plenty of flesh.

(b) I have small bones and overall well balanced body.
(c) I have average sized bones and am solidly built with good muscular development.

6. Which of the following best describes your chest and shoulder regions?
(a) It is large and wide but flabby with excess flesh.
(b) It is weak, sloping and sunken, and is the weakest region of my body.
(c) It is wide, strong and well developed, and is the most developed region of my body.
(d) It is wide and solid.
7. Which of the following foods do you prefer the most?
(a) Hot foods
(b) Warm foods
(c) Cool foods
(d) Cold foods
8. In general, your hands and/or feet are:
(a) Generally cold
(b) Generally warm
9. How would you describe your manner of walking?
(a) My pace is generally slow with a measured gait and a dignified appearance
(b) I tend to walk carefully but on the whole it is natural and gentle.
(c) I walk with a light and fast tempo, and have a tendency to shake my body (people say it is not stable).
(d) I walk with a very straight and stiff posture, at times resembling the walk of a robot.
10. In general, which of the following best describes how you sweat and your feeling after sweating?
(a) I usually sweat a lot and feel invigorated after sweating.
(b) I usually do not sweat much and feel tired even after sweating just a little.
(c) I usually do not feel tired after sweating.
11. Do your hands easily chap during winter?
(a) Yes
(b) No
12. Which of the following best describe your personality?
(a) I never hesitate and am resolute.
(b) I am very active and brave.

(c) I have a dignified appearance and am formal.
(d) I have gentle and frank manners.

13. Which of the following best describes your inner nature?
    (a) I frequently take other's thoughts and accomplishments as my own.
    (b) I frequently despise others.
    (c) I frequently hear that I am greedy.
    (d) I frequently hear that I am jealous and envious.
14. Which of the following best describes you?
    (a) I do not like people who are overly courteous.
    (b) I do not like people who act in overly dignified manner.
    (c) I do not like people who are overly righteous.
    (d) I do not like people who think that they know it all.
15. Which of the following best describes you?
    (a) No matter what work I am involved in, I push forward without backing up.
    (b) I tend to start projects easily but have problems finishing them.
    (c) I tend to push forth with the work quietly by myself.
    (d) I tend to stay in one location and do not tend to go out.

B Carefully read the questions on the following sections and check the ones that best describe you on the answer sheet. If the question does not belong to you, leave the space blank.

- **Your Work Performance and Your Strengths and Weaknesses**

16. Rather than working at a salary job for someone else, I would rather work for myself as an independent contractor even though my income would be somewhat inconsistent.
17. No matter what projects or work I am given, I quickly take care of them.
18. I am comfortable getting acquainted with or making new friends.
19. I am active and strong willed.
20. I tend to start or enter into every affair without much thought as to the pros and cons.
21. No matter how difficult the task is, I always accomplish what I start out to do.
22. I can patiently stay and work in one location for a long time
23. I tend to be very precise and meticulous in all my affairs.
24. I tend to socialize only with those whom I am close to.
25. I can easily make friends without considering pros and cons.

26. I focus more on social affairs than on my own work.
27. I focus more on my own work than to social affairs.
28. I put more emphasis on my appearance than on my inner self.
29. I put more emphasis on my inner self more so than to my appearance.
30. I tend to be very picky when it comes to making friends, so forming friendships does not come easily to me.
31. I am very quick in action and I am courageous.
32. No matter what the work, I do it very thoroughly.
33. I have a proper and prudent personality.
34. I tend to be very active and I am straightforward in all matters.

- **Personal Relationship**

35. I tend to be extremely tolerant and understanding of others.
36. I tend to exercise moderation and am generally conservative.
37. I am very good at teaching others and can be quite persuasive when I want to be.
38. My passion and empathy makes it easy for me to soothe people.
39. I enjoy participating in various social activities.

- **When I See a Person:**

40. I can quickly sense whether or not he/she is the right person for the job.
41. I can quickly sense whether or not he/she is an honest person.
42. I first seek to find out his/her educational level.
43. I can quickly sense whether or not he/she is smart.
44. I can quickly sense whether or not he/she is diligent.
45. I can quickly sense whether or not he/she is sincere.
46. I first seek to sense his/her ability or talent.
47. I can quickly sense whether or not he/she is capable.

- **General Mental Attitude**

48. I tend to always hurry things.
49. I am always anxious since I always start projects but seldom finish them.
50. I have difficulty facing an audience for the first time.
51. I am usually timid and often feel insecure.
52. I am usually very sensitive emotionally.
53. I have great patience and/or perseverance.
54. I often embellish stories I tell

55. I tend to act hastily (rashly).
56. I hold grudges for a long time.
57. I tend to work according to my moods and feelings.
58. I become quickly bored and give up easily on everything that I do.
59. I feel congestion in my chest when I think of the many things that I have to take care of.
60. I tend toward masculine characteristics such as machismo, heroic deeds, chivalry and athletics more so than feminine qualities such as gentility, kindness and love.

• Personal Problems

61. Though I know many people, I really do not have any close friends.
62. I tend to go out a lot and as a result often neglect managing family affairs, housework or chores.
63. I have difficulty easily adapting to new work or environment.
64. I frequently get distressed over my difficulty in making friends.
65. I get annoyed over trivial things.
66. I have difficulty speaking or making a presentation before an audience.

• Emotional Characteristics

67. I become livid with anger if I am looked down upon or taken lightly.
68. I am usually cheerful but my emotions tend to fluctuate greatly.
69. Though my feelings are hurt, I pretend that I am fine.
70. Though I usually do not try to stand out in a crowd, inwardly, I wish everyone would take notice of me.
71. I frequently feel annoyed, restless and anxious.

• Behavioral Characteristic

72. I do not speak indiscriminately until I feel certain that my ideas are correct.
73. I frequently act and behave without courtesy towards others.
74. I frequently pretend that I know it all or show off.
75. I pretend to be modest by not showing what I have.
76. I am unconcerned about other people's business and do not want to be bothered by others in my own business.
77. I tend to do as I please without being concerned about other

people's thoughts or feelings.

78. In every undertaking or business affair, I am usually tactful and proficient.
79. I frequently pretend to be well behaved.
80. I often make excuses to skip a party, gathering or meeting.
81. While at work, I can do a good job even though my surroundings are noisy.
82. I put more enthusiasm into the work of others compared to my own.
83. Though I want to be recognized or acknowledged, I tend to be indifferent toward others.
84. I treat others with more respect than I treat myself.
85. I usually like to receive rewards but have difficulty rewarding others.
86. People generally come to me when they need to persuade others.
87. I am uncomfortable appearing before others.
88. I am so timid that I frequently feel anxious, uneasy or insecure.
89. I often have the desire to make someone else's ideas and achievements my own.
90. I am often jealous over other people's possessions.
91. I am not very courteous or polite toward others.
92. I tend to neglect domestic chores.
93. I am usually indifferent to affairs that are not my own.
94. I tend to shrink from danger in all affairs.
95. In speech, I say let us open our hearts and be open and free, yet in action, I am just the opposite.
96. Even though I have accomplished something considerable, I often feel something remains lacking.
97. Even though I am diligent in doing other people's work, I frequently feel that I am not doing enough for them.
98. Even though I have most things I need, I still often feel something is lacking.
99. I often feel joyful even in trivial matters.
100. I have more feminine aspects that the masculine aspect.

- **Physical Condition**

101. I have, at times, without any reason, vomited or had difficulty swallowing foods and drinks.
102. I often have the feeling of not being relieved after a bowel movement with a desire to go back to the bathroom.

103. I tend toward constipation and it is usually unbearable.
104. When I have chronic diarrhea, my lower abdomen feels cold.
105. I often feel as if my body is getting well after I have started to sweat in the palms of my hands and soles of my feet.
106. I often feel as if my body is getting well after I have started to sweat in the area between the top of my lip and the bottom of my nose.
107. When I get sick, the first thing I experience is difficulty in urination.
108. I have a tendency to get constipated when I get sick.
109. I feel better when I sweat during an illness.
110. When I get sick, the first thing I experience is indigestion.
111. I sigh often because I generally do not have much energy.
112. I have difficulty in moving around due to loss of energy in my body and legs.
113. I often have a distended sensation in my chest and abdomen after meals.
114. Even when I am in a healthy condition, I often experience palpitations.
115. Frequently, my arms and legs feel weak and my hands and feet tremble.
116. Sometimes, my eyes are sore and/or get red easily.
117. I feel a dry and rough sensation around my eyes at times.
118. I sometimes experience a stifling, painful sensation in my chest.
119. Even though I usually sweat very little, I have had occasions where I have broken into a cold sweat as my illness got worse.
120. I sweat a great deal even when I eat cold foods in the winter.

Tallying up the Scores

The answer sheet for these questions and the number related to each constitution can be found at the end of this book.

Taking this test is simple. First of all, questions one to 15 are multiple choices, so select the answers that pertain to you and mark them on the answer sheet. From questions 16 to 121, answer only those that directly pertain to you. Then, study the Sasang criterion on the reverse side of the answer sheet and count the total number of constitutional criterion. For example, if *Taeyangin* criterion is two, *Soyangin* criterion is four, *Tae-eumin* criterion is 25 and *Soeumin* criterion is 10, you are *Tae-eumin* constitution.

If there is no predominant criterion, it is hard to differentiate your constitution through this test. Therefore, it is recommended that you consult with an SCM specialist.

Even though this questionnaire is a simple method of differentiating constitution, there are some drawbacks to its use. One of the problems is that all the questions have equal weight. That is, the test fails to emphasize those questions that are more important in distinguishing the constitution in relation to those that are less important.

Another problem is that it is difficult to fairly and objectively evaluate one's own life. One way to solve this problem is to ask a close family member to answer the questions after you have finished them and then compare the two sets of answers.

The constitutional assessment test is the easiest way to determine one's constitution and the majority of the readers should be able to determine their own constitution. However, the accuracy of the constitutional assessment test depends on the following factors: environment, cultivation of the mind and truthfulness of the answers.

Reference

Body Measuring Method: Using a Ruler to Take Body Measurements in order to Determine the Constitution

Dr. Lee Je-ma book, *Longevity and Life Preservation in Eastern Medicine,* presents the theory that there are developed regions and weak regions in each constitution. The book states, "*Taeyangins* have a developed Upper Burner but a weak Lower-Middle Burner. *Soyangins* have a developed Upper-Middle Burner but a weak Lower Burner. *Tae-eumins* have a developed Lower-Middle Burner but a weak Upper Burner. *Soeumins* have a developed Lower Burner but a weak Upper-Middle Burner." The measuring method to determine constitution was created based on this theory.

Dr. Huh Man-hoi bases the measuring method presented here on a research paper. This method established five standardized measurement lines based on "A Discourse on Viscera and Bowels" discussed in *Longevity and Life Preservation in Eastern Medicine* as well as morphological configuration based on "A Discourse on Four Principles" and "A Discourse on Establishment and Supplement" of the same book.

When the body shape of each constitution is drawn into a figure, they are as follows:

1. Four Male Constitutions

Taeyangin 태양인

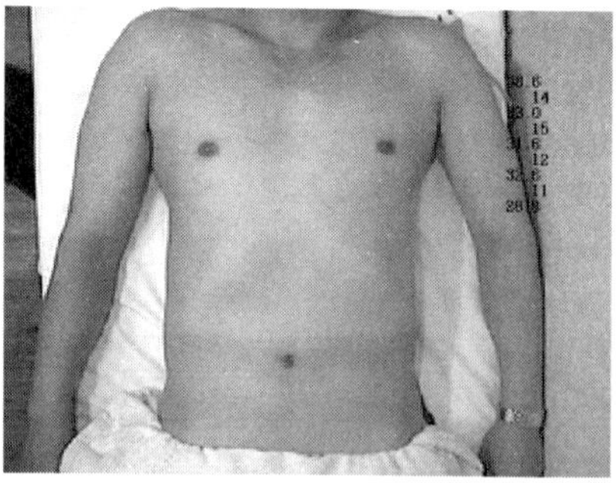

Tae-eumin 태음인

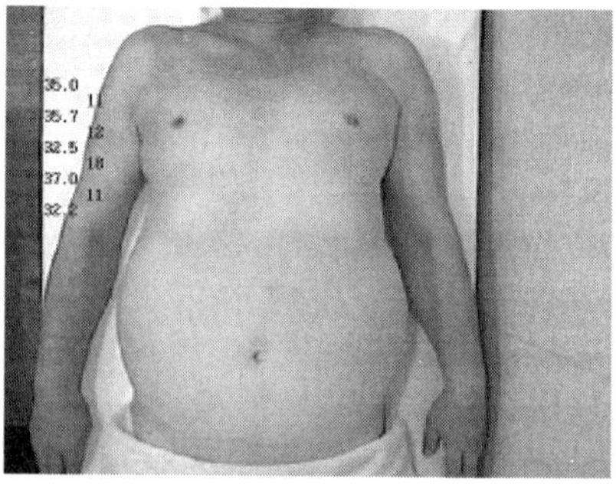

Soyangin 소양인

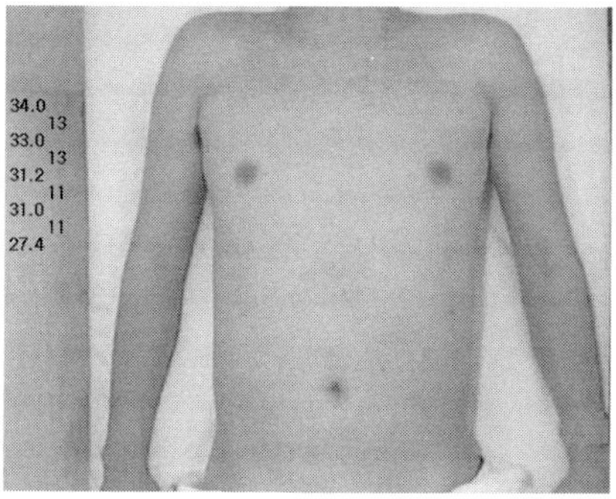

Soeumin 소음인

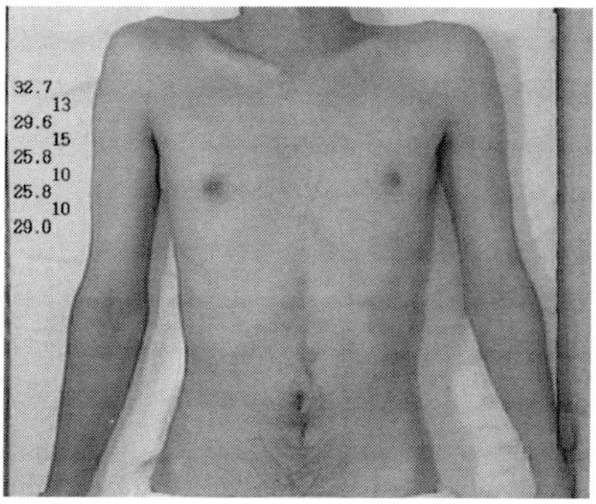

2. Four Female Constitutions

Taeyangin 태양인

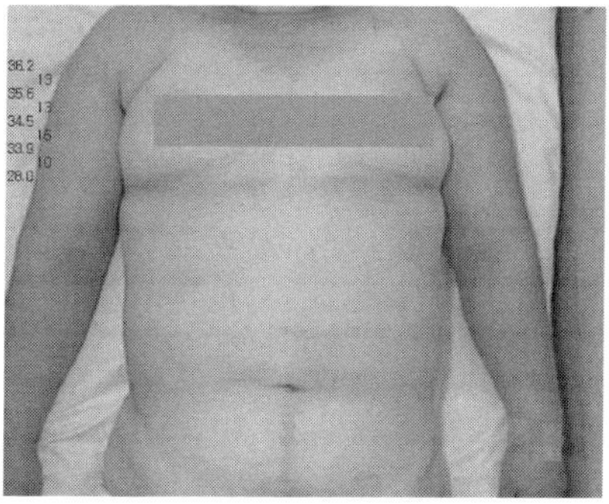

Tae-eumin 태음인

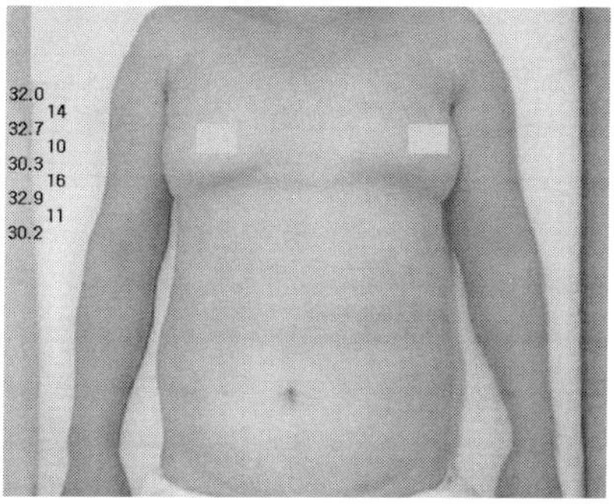

Soyangin 소양인

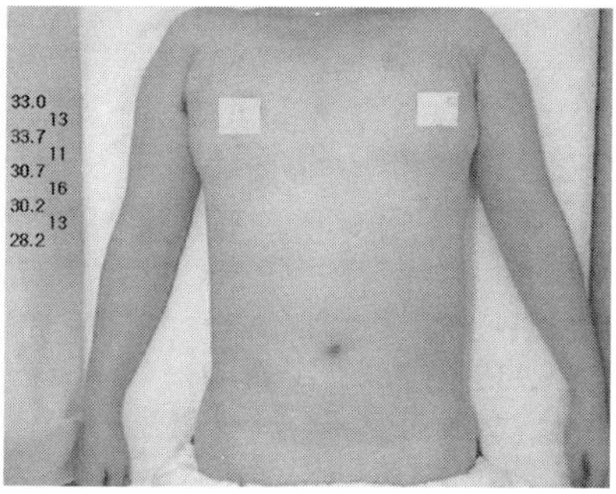

Soeumin 소음인

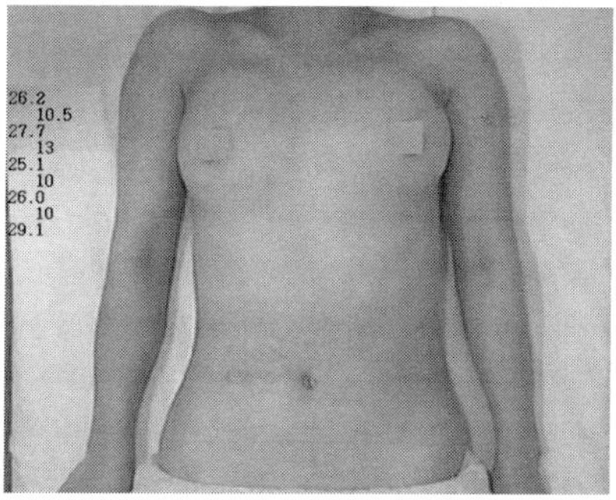

The five standardized measurement lines that are based on "A Discourse on Viscera and Bowels" are as follows:

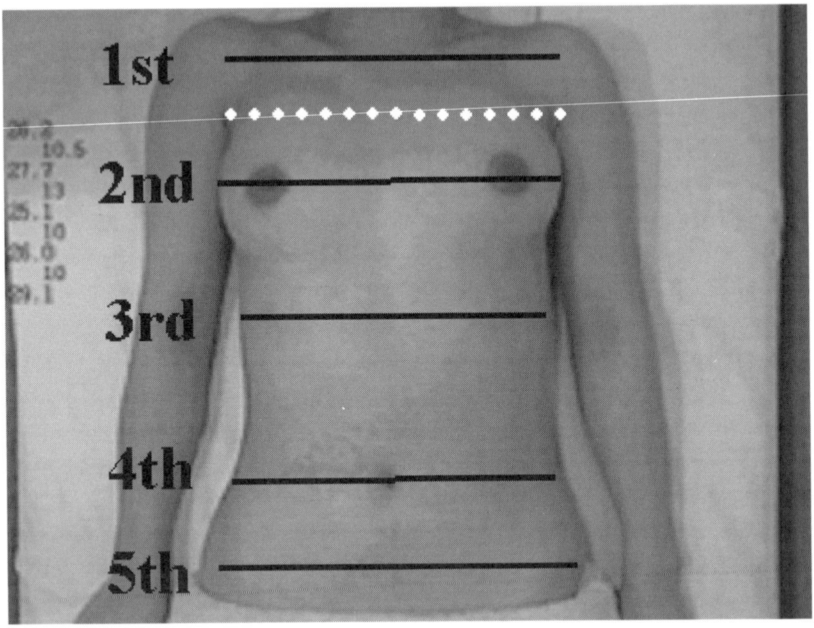

Five Standardized Measurement Lines

1. The first line (shoulder region)-the length of the horizontal line connecting the left and right axillary folds which are on the superolateral aspect of the pectoralis major muscle.
   Originally the first line should be measured by checking the distance of Rt. & Lt. hollow portions between the acromion and the coracoid process. However, it's easy to make mistakes in measuring the first line. That's why how to check the first line is changed into measuring the distance between Rt. & Lt axillary folds at the beginning points. The dotted line is where you will measure the first line.

* Axillary fold: the depressed area on both armpits.

* Pectoralis major muscle: the chest muscle that has a triangular shape. This muscle moves with movement of the arm or breathing.

2. The second line (chest region)-the length of the horizontal line crossing both nipples and reaching Rt. & Lt. lateral sides.
3. The third line (stomach region)-the length of the horizontal line crossing both ST-19 points and reaching Rt. & Lt. lateral sides passing through Rt. & Lt. protruded portions of the mixed cartilages of 7th and 8th ribs.

* ST-19: 6 cuns above the umbilicus, 2 cuns lateral to the REN-14.

4. The fourth line (umbilicus area)-the length of the horizontal line crossing both ST-25 points passing through the navel and reaching Rt. & Lt. lateral sides.

* ST-25: 2 cuns lateral to the center of umbilicus.

5. The 5th line (ilium area)-the length of the horizontal line reaching both lateral sides of the left and right anterior superior iliac spine.

* Ilium: The region where the belt is hung when wearing pants.

Based on this, the five standard measurement lines were named the shoulder line (standard line for Upper Burner), the chest line (standard line for Upper-Middle Burner), the stomach line (line for dividing *yin* and *yang*), the umbilical line (standard line for Lower-Middle Burner), and the ilium line (standard line for Lower Burner). Those five standard measurement lines, measured, three hundred and eleven people whose constitutions were ascertained based on clinical findings and the results of the statistics were as follows:

Average Length Per Region

(Unit in cm. /Round off fraction to two decimal places)

	Taeyangin	*Soyangin*	*Tae-eumin*	*Soeumin*
Shoulder region	35.6 34.9-36.3)	30.3 (28.9-31.6)	27.7 (27.0-28.3)	26.5 (26.2-26.8)
Chest region	31.9 (31.0-32.8)	27.9 (26.7-29.1)	30.1 (29.4-30.8)	28.8 (28.4-29.2)
Stomach region	30.5 (29.6-31.4)	26.4 (25.3-27.6)	29.7 (29.1-30.3)	27.0 (26.6-27.4)
Navel region	28.6 (27.5-29.8)	25.0 (23.8-26.1)	30.2 (29.5-30.9)	28.1 (27.6-28.6)
Hip bone (ASIS)	25.3 (24.6-25.9)	23.9 (22.7-25.1)	27.5 (26.8-28.2)	29.9 (29.4-30.3)

This research found the particular characteristics of each constitution by dividing the trunk into Four Burners based on the Theory of Four Burners in *Longevity and Life Preservation in Eastern Medicine* and measuring the five standard measurement lines that are the landmarks of the four burners.

When the results were reviewed, *Soeumins* showed a clear

weakness of the upper body. The depression of first line is clear, while the fifth line is long so that the anterior superior iliac spine clearly protrudes outward. In addition, the pelvis is spread wider than those of the other constitutions. The measurements for the third and fourth lines, meanwhile, are short so that the Lower-Middle Burner is depressed inward, similar to an hourglass figure.

Soyangins are the constitution in which the Upper-Middle Burner is well developed. Elasticity of the pectoralis major muscle is felt and the measurements from the first line to fifth line show gradual narrowing so that the first line is the longest and the fifth line is the shortest.

Tae-eumins have a weaker upper body while the abdominal region, which is the Lower-Middle Burner, is the most developed. Thus, the measurement of the fourth line is the longest in relation to other constitutions. The third and the fifth lines are either the same or the fifth line is one to two centimeters shorter than the third line.

The first line in *Taeyangins* is generally longer than 36 centimeters and there is a difference of at least 10 centimeters or greater between the first and fifth line. There is a gradual narrowing from the first to the fifth line.

This is a corroborative method that validates the particulars of constitutional morphology by fixed diagnostic index after establishing the hypothesis based on the *Longevity and Life Preservation in Eastern Medicine*.

Getting a total picture of a person is important no matter what type of diagnostic method is used. Therefore, since this diagnostic method emphasizes the particulars of external physical measurement of each constitution, other factors such as the nature of the mind and disease symptoms must be considered as well.

This method is simple, convenient, objective and is based on standardized measurements. It is reproducible and can be objectively verified by obtaining the measurement using this technique. Therefore, it is one of the most important diagnostic methods to accurately differentiate constitutions.

Chapter 3
Daily Health Maintenance Using Sasang Constitutional Theory

Everyone should have been able to roughly identify their own constitution after reading the previous chapter. Let us now think about how we can apply the information.

In each constitution, there are certain emotions that warrant caution and certain principles to regulate these emotions. There are certain foods that are to be avoided and foods that are appropriate. There are herbs that are either beneficial or harmful to one's constitution, and there are certain principles to treat diseases as well as rules for longevity that allow a person to acquire lifelong health.

Knowing one's constitution is not only helpful for physical health but also for harmonious social and family life. This is because each constitution has different characteristics which allow one to recognize his or her abilities and temperament as well as the merits and demerits of one's personality. Through such means, one can regulate one's mind and behavior, and thus maintain a healthy mind and body. Additionally, by knowing which things to be aware of, a person can confidently deal with everyday affairs. One's understanding of others will also deepen so that one can develop the good habit of giving warm consideration to others, leading to better overall relationships.

Clearly there are many things to be gained through understanding constitutions. This chapter contains health cultivation methods that are readily applicable to daily life.

1. Beneficial or Harmful Foods

Traditionally it is said that food and medicine have the same origin. This implies that diet is just as important as medicine in the treatment and prevention of disease.

As foods have less of an energetic variance than medicine, it can be said that they act more mildly on the body. It is clear, however, that there are beneficial and harmful foods according to each constitution. Nevertheless, since foods are taken for a long period of time, they are even more important than medicine. Foods that are appropriate for the constitution are the best tonic, but those that are inappropriate will become toxins that gradually accumulate in the body and cause disease.

Eating foods that are appropriate for the constitution will suppress the strength of organs that have excessive energy and will strengthen organs that are deficient. This will result in a harmonious balance. *Yang* types will be induced to *yin* tendencies and *yin* types will be induced to *yang* tendencies so that both types can achieve balance.

What vegetables make the best morning juice? What kind of fruits will be good to us? What tonics are the best? Is there any food that is especially harmful? Are there certain guidelines to follow as a fundamental principle in selecting proper foods? These are questions that people frequently ask.

Some foods supply energy while others have a medicinal effect. Both of these actions are taken into consideration in SCM. This encourages us to be scrupulous in the selection of daily foods and to better understand those foods that supplement our constitutional weaknesses or imbalances.

This does not mean that you cannot eat foods that are inappropriate for your constitution. It only means that you should eat more foods that are appropriate for your constitution. For instance, if you want to add a special health food to your diet, it should be selected from the foods recognized by SCM to benefit your particular constitution. Your diet should also be regulated if you habitually over-eat foods inappropriate for your constitution.

Many people in their middle and older years attempt to supplement their diets with vegetable juices or mixtures of eggs, apples and oranges. They do this because they feel that there is something lacking in their diet. They believe that their health will improve if they change or supplement their usual diet. The real question is, however, what determines the standard by which proper foods are selected.

One example is that many people eat chicken because it is known to have high nutritional value. In Korea, chicken soup made with ginseng is popular as a summertime nutritional boost. Unfortunately, *Soyangins* need to avoid this kind of soup; in severe cases they can develop skin rashes and red eyes. Even if a *Soyangin* does not have these adverse reactions, he or she is still recommended not to eat chicken or take ginseng as a tonic for an extended period of time. Western medicine would attribute these symptoms to allergic reactions, but SCM systematically explains the method of selecting the correct foods for each constitution.

Western medicine uses diet therapy as well. Patients with abnormal liver functions, for example, are advised to eat foods that are high in protein and low in fat. They are advised to ingest large amounts of fish, including shellfish. Thus, the dietary measures in western medicine vary depending on a patient's condition. SCM uses the diet in a different way. It does not deal with specific diseases per se, instead it discusses the proper method to regulate and balance one's constitution.

In general, cold foods and drinks are not appropriate for *yin* types while warm foods and drinks are not appropriate for *yang* types. People who develop abdominal pain and/or diarrhea after ingesting many cold summer fruits, like watermelon, muskmelon, or cold drinks, like draft beers or soft drinks, are generally *Soeumins*. Since they have weak digestive systems and cold bodies, foods that are cold or hard to digest are not good for them. On the contrary, foods that are easy to digest or warm, like chicken, are appropriate for them and can warm up their cold bodies.

When preparing foods, *Soeumins* are advised to use stimulating condiments to help increase the appetite and digestion and to avoid using large amounts of oil or eating bland food. *Soeumins* should develop a habit of enjoying warm drinks or foods. Even in summer, it is better to drink warm water than to drink ice cold water.

Soyangins have a good digestive system, so they digest all kinds of food easily. Even in winter, they have no troubles with cold foods like cold buckwheat noodles or cold drinks. Parents of *Soyangin* children do not need to worry even if their child enjoys eating ice cream in the winter. Though there may be a concern for tooth decay, it is rare that *Soyangins* develop digestive problems from eating ice cream.

Soyangins do not usually have trouble selecting foods. They are not fussy eaters and have a good appetite and good digestion. But since they have a great deal of heat in their constitution, they must carefully avoid foods that induce heat in the body. Foods that are appropriate for *Soeumins*, such as chicken and honey, are actually not beneficial for *Soyangins*.

Since the question of digestion is not a concern for *Soyangins*, they should select foods based on their temperature. Because *Soyangins* easily develop a deficiency of *yin*, foods that have the ability to nourish *yin* are recommended. In terms of grains and legumes, barley, aduki beans, and mung beans are best for them.

Like the *Soyangins*, *Taeyangins* are also advised to ingest fresh, cold foods. The difference is that *Soyangins* have a vigorous digestive function that can handle fatty foods, whereas *Taeyangins* are better suited with plain foods. Foods that are low in fat and bland foods without added spices are appropriate for *Taeyangins*.

Since *Taeyangins* have a weak Liver function, if they regularly ingest foods high in calories and high in protein, which can overburden the Liver, they can develop Liver problems.

Tae-eumins have a weak Upper Burner and so are

susceptible to respiratory and circulatory system disorders. They are usually overweight and thus should avoid foods with high cholesterol that are known to cause heart disease or stroke. Also they are encouraged to ingest foods which can strengthen their weak Lung function.

For them, foods that are rich in protein are recommended instead of fatty foods. But as they have the habit of overeating, *Tae-eumins* are susceptible to obesity, hypertension and constipation. Thus they must avoid foods that are stimulating and fatty. Moreover, they should avoid over eating even the foods appropriate to their constitution and exercise regularly or take saunas to promote sweating and prevent obesity. It is also important for *Tae-eumins* to keep proper dietary measures by eating foods with fiber to eliminate habitual constipation.

The following is a list of grains, meats, seafood, vegetables and fruits that are appropriate for each constitution:

1) *Taeyangin*

For *Taeyangins*, foods that are plain or bland or foods that strengthen the Liver and nourish *yin* are appropriate. Seafood and vegetables, which are low in fat, are especially good.

- Grains: buckwheat
- Seafood: shrimp, oyster, abalone, wreath shell, crab, sea cucumber, crucian carp
- Vegetables: water shield plant, pine needles
- Fruits: grapes, wild grapes, Asian kiwi, persimmons, cherries, Chinese quince, pine pollen

* Harmful Foods: those that are pungent, hot, spicy or greasy

2) *Soyangin*

Since *Soyangins* have a lot of heat in their bodies, seafood, vegetables and foods that are fresh and cold are beneficial. Since their bodies can easily develop *yin* deficiency, foods that nourish *yin* are good.

- Grains/legumes: barley, aduki beans, and mung beans
- Meat/poultry: pork, duck
- Seafood: oyster, sea cucumber, sea squirt, abalone, shrimp, crab, globefish, lobster, carp, northern snake-head fish, tortoise, and flatfish
- Vegetables: Chinese cabbage, cucumber, lettuce, burdock, and eggplant
- Fruits: watermelon, muskmelon, strawberries, bananas, and pineapple
- Others: beer, iced drinks

* Harmful foods: pungent, stimulating condiments such as hot pepper, ginger, green onion, garlic, mustard, curry, chicken, goat meat, honey, and ginseng

3) *Tae-eumin*

Tae-eumins generally have large bodies and a good digestive system. Thus they are recommended to ingest foods that are high in either animal or vegetable protein.

- Grains/legumes: wheat, beans, yams, job's tear, millet, peanuts, perilla seeds, sugar, and brown rice
- Meat/poultry: beef, milk, butter, and cheese
- Seafood: cod liver oil, spawn of Pollack, mud snail, eel, cod, brown seaweed, kelp, and laver
- Fruits/nuts: chestnuts, pine nuts, walnuts, gingko nuts, pear, maesil (Japanese apricot), apricot, and plums
- Vegetables: radishes, broad bellflower, carrots, glehnia root, braken, lotus roots, taro, yams, and mushrooms

* Harmful foods: chicken, pork, ginseng, honey, and ginger

4) *Soeumin*

Since *Soeumins* can easily develop stomach disturbances due to a weak digestive system, spices and warm foods are good for them. Fatty foods, cold foods and raw foods can easily cause diarrhea.

- Grains: glutinous rice, glutinous millet, and potatoes
- Fruits: apples, oranges, tomatoes, peaches, and jujubes
- Meat/poultry: chicken, deer meat, sparrow, pheasant, goat's milk, goat, lamb, and honey
- Seafood: Alaskan Pollack, red snapper, anchovy, croaker, and mud snail
- Vegetables: spinach, cabbage, dropwort, green onion, garlic, ginger, red pepper, mustard, black pepper, and curry

* Harmful foods: cold noodles, muskmelon, watermelon, cold milk, ice cream, beer, barley, pork, cuttlefish, and wheat products

2. Teas

Today many people in Korea prefer western style drinks, like cocoa or coffee, to traditional teas. This is probably due to the fact that they are easily accessible from vending machines. It is also because of a blind liking for anything western civilization has to offer.

It is wonderful to see that recently people have begun to return to traditional teas in consideration of their health. However, since not all teas are beneficial for everyone, it is important to drink the teas that match your constitution.

According to personal preferences, people enjoy a wide variety of tastes such as pungent, sweet, bitter, savory, sour, etc. When choosing a tea, try to prepare and drink at home or work the tea that matches your taste preference and has the energetic nature that complements your constitution.

Tea made from the Chinese quince is most appropriate for *Taeyangins*. Its sour and bitter tastes relate well with their constitution. Chinese quince is good for those *Taeyangins* who lack energy, are fatigued and have no desires in their daily lives. This tea also helps treat indigestion or headaches that are stress related. Other teas that are good for *Taeyangins* include persimmon leaf or acanthopanax[4].

Lycium fruit[5] tea is good for *Soyangins*. Lycium has a sweet and slightly bitter taste that may be somewhat offensive for first-timers. For *Soyangins*, pineapple juice or green vegetable juice is actually better than hot teas. Hot teas made from ginseng or honey and the *Ssanghwa* tea (Double Harmony tea), which is a combination of herbs such as rehmannia, peony, cinnamon, licorice and Chinese angelica, should be avoided.

Teas made from the green perilla leaf, Job's tear, and kudzu are good for *Tae-eumins*. The Job's tear tea generally sold in stores is a combination of both Job's tear and green perilla, so it is an appropriate tea for the *Tae-eumin* constitution. The pharmacological name of kudzu[6] tea is radix puerariae. It is somewhat bitter and somewhat sweet. It can reduce the fever by promoting sweating, so it is frequently found in formulas that treat the common cold or flu. It can be taken as a hot tea or extracted into a fresh juice. The fresh juice is also effective for hangovers.

There are many varieties of teas appropriate for *Soeumins*. Some examples include cinnamon tea, ginseng tea, fresh ginger tea, honey tea and the *ssanghwa* tea (Double Harmony tea).

Px

Drinking cinnamon tea in the winter can prevent colds because it can promote sweating and remove the coldness in the body. Five to six servings of cinnamon tea can be prepared by boiling 15 grams of cinnamon, five to ten pieces of Chinese red dates and three grams of fresh ginger together. A little honey or

---

4) root bark of various araliaceous shrubs.

5) the dried fruit of the Chinese matrimony vine.

6) arrowroot.

sugar can also be added according to individual preferences. Ginseng tea can be bought pre-packaged in the supermarket or it can be made by combining white ginseng or fresh ginseng with jujubes and a little honey.

3. Constitutions and Diseases

There are many ways to treat a disease. We frequently see that one treatment method is effective for one person but not for another. There is no one "cure-all" treatment method that can be used for all people. Instead the treatment method must change from person to person, and constitution to constitution.

It is a misinterpretation of the term "improving the constitution" that has allowed people to think that constitutions can change over time. Constitutions do not change over time, but the mind does change over time.

SCM has three fundamental principles. The first is that constitutions do not change over time. Secondly, it states that there are only the four constitutional types. The third principle is that herbal medicines are only used according to the patient's constitution. These three principles are strictly followed in SCM.

There are uniform patterns of physiology, pathology and psychology that manifest according to each constitution. Thus, applying the particular characteristics of herbal medicines or foods to supplement the constitutions is the most effective treatment method whether treating diseases or improving a weak constitution .

The methods of health cultivation through dietary guidelines and the regulation of one's mind and body according to SCM principles can be easily understood and applied by lay persons. However, differentiating disease patterns according to the constitutions and assessing disease progression and prognosis as well as applying accurate herbal formulas should be left to SCM specialists.

1) *Taeyangin*

Taeyangins are healthy when they urinate with ease and in great amounts. When there is any new problem with urination, one must first suspect an illness.

If *Taeyangins* over-eat hot, spicy, or greasy foods rather than raw or cool foods, they can develop disease in the esophagus or stomach region. In general *Taeyangins* dislike standing or walking for a long period of time because of their inherent lower body weakness. Thus if they do not exercise their lower bodies, they are susceptible to developing diseases in that region. Also if they become emotional and get easily angered or retain grief for a long time, they can easily develop diseases in the Liver region.

The constitutional disease syndromes of *Taeyangins* include *yul-gyuk* (dysphagia), *ban-wyi* (vomiting), and *hae-yuk* (lower body weakness). These syndromes, however, do not appear unless the symptoms are serious. In the *yul-gyuk* syndrome there is a difficulty in swallowing food and even the food that is swallowed does not reach the stomach as it is vomited out. During this syndrome the esophageal region feels as though there is cool air running through it. When this symptom appears, the disease is considered to be serious. The situation is urgent and in need of immediate attention. If, however, the person has a high fever and pain in the body or abdomen, or has gurgling sounds in the abdomen with diarrhea or dysentery, it is not *yul-gyuk* (dysphagia) syndrome.

In the *ban-wyi* (vomiting) syndrome, there is no problem in swallowing food, but after eating the epigastric region feels full and uncomfortable and after several hours the food is vomited up. It is said that food eaten in the morning is vomited up in the evening and food eaten in the evening is vomited up the next morning. In terms of western medicine, these symptoms are seen in diseases such as stomach cancer, atony of the stomach,* and pyloric stenosis.

In the *hae-yuk* (lower body weakness) syndrome, there is

* also Gastroparesis?

severe fatigue and a weakness of the lower body and legs so that even walking is uncomfortable. However, there is no paralysis, swelling or pain, and no chills or fever. This syndrome occurs due to a disease in the spine rather than a direct weakness of the legs.

In addition to copious and unobstructed urination, *Taeyangins* are considered healthy when their bowel movements are easy and contain many large stools. A pale complexion is a sign of health, while a dark complexion is not. It is better for this constitution to be thin rather than obese. It is also not good if a solid mass develops in the epigastric region. If the mass is small, the disease is mild but if it is large, the disease is serious.

As previously stated, the pathology and the pharmacology of the *Taeyangins* are not well known. Dr. Lee Je-ma mentioned a few individual herbs and two formulas that are suitable for this constitution. Currently, the doctors who studied SCM after the passing of Dr. Lee Je-ma say that *Taeyangins* easily develop diseases and symptoms such as liver disease, indigestion, esophageal stenosis, esophageal cancer, stomach cancer, heat sensation rising in the head, weakness of legs, and eye disorders. They are also seeking to develop and research new formulas to be applied for those with *Taeyangin* constitution.

2) *Soyangin*

Soyangins are healthy when they have regular bowel movements. Even if there is a slight disease condition, under these circumstances it will soon disappear. In contrast, a disease should be suspected when there is any problem with bowel movements, even if there are no other symptoms. If there is no bowel movement for two to three days and the person has fullness and a painful sensation in the chest that is unbearable, it is a sign of serious disease and must be treated immediately.

It is a particular characteristic of *Soyangins* to have a heat sensation in the chest when they have chronic constipation. This is due to pathogenic heat that stagnates in the chest region instead of descending and being eliminated.

Soyangins have weak urinary and reproductive systems so they easily develop problems in the organs associated with excretion, such as the bladder or kidneys. As *Soyangins* have weakness in their waist and legs, they frequently suffer from low back pain due to problems in the spine or hip joint. They are susceptible to summer heat because they have a lot of heat in their bodies. At times, they develop skin rashes when they eat foods that do not match their constitution.

Since *Soyangins*' digestive system is good when they are in a balanced state, they are not hindered by any foods and rarely develop stomach diseases. But they must be careful not to eat too quickly for they are impatient.

The progression of disease in a *yin* constitution is slow. Both the progression and the healing of a disease take time. A disease does not worsen quickly nor do *yin* constitutions easily recover from a disease once it has started. In contrast, the progression and disappearance of diseases in *yang* types is rapid. A disease can be readily aggravated but it can also improve quickly once healing begins. Because disease symptoms in *Soyangins* are due to Fire and Heat, the progression of the disease is rapid and warrants caution even in its initial stage. *Soyangins* must be attentive, especially if there are headaches or constipations that accompany an illness.

The most important thing to understand about *Soyangin's* disease is the condition of the bowel movements. Their stool should initially come out dry and the latter part should be loose and easily eliminated. It is a sign that they are recovering from an illness if they eliminate large amounts of loose stool once or twice and then no more. Having loose stool once or twice a day does not indicate the worsening of disease. If, however, there is an absence of bowel movements for more than one day or slight diarrhea three to five times in a day, it is a sign that there will be constipation in the near future, which does not bode well.

Intermittent nose bleeding or blood in the saliva or phlegm

in *Soyangins* is considered to be the vomiting of blood even if it is in small amounts. Also, cold saliva coming up inside the mouth is considered vomiting as well, even though there is no actual vomiting of food or water. These two symptoms, vomiting blood and vomiting, are indications of a serious disease in *Soyangins* and must be treated immediately. Moreover, as the progression of edema is quick in *Soyangins*, it must also be treated immediately.

In *Soyangins*, sweating from the soles and palms is a sign of healing. However, if there is an absence of sweating from the palms and soles of their feet, the disease will not heal even if there is sweating all over the rest of the body.

Since the pathology and pharmacology of *Soyangins* are fairly well known, applying constitutional medicine for them is simple.

3) *Tae-eumin*

Tae-eumins are healthy when they sweat easily. We often think that profuse sweating is a symptom of a weakened bodily condition. But in *Tae-eumins*, it is a proof that they are healthy, so we need not worry. When *Tae-eumins* feel uncomfortable, exercising and bathing to induce sweating will refresh them. In contrast, if there is an absence of sweating, one must suspect a possible illness. It is almost certain that a disease is in progress if their pores are closed and they cannot sweat.

Tae-eumins can easily develop diseases such as heart disease, hypertension, stroke, bronchitis, and asthma due to a weakness in their respiratory and circulatory systems. They must also be cautious of skin diseases such as eczema and rashes and other diseases such as enteritis, hemorrhoids and neurosis.

Soyangins can immediately burn up whatever they've eaten, but *Tae-eumins* are relatively inactive in relation to the large amounts of food that they ingest. So they are susceptible to obesity and constipation. They must develop a daily exercise routine to induce sweating and to prevent obesity. They must also maintain good dietary habits to prevent constipation.

Tae-eumins are easily afflicted with blood stagnation in the Liver, which creates heat and causes the stool to dry up.

Although constipation occurs frequently in *Tae-eumins*, it is not a significant problem. It is a sign of a serious illness, however, when there is chronic diarrhea with a sensation of fog clogging up the Lower-Middle Burner of the Small Intestines.

The color of the complexion can also be used to distinguish the severity of an illness. If *Tae-eumins* have a pale bluish color to their complexion, there is not much dryness and heat, but if the complexion is yellow or dark red, there is much heat in the Liver and much dryness in the Lungs.

The treatment principle of *Tae-eumins'* diseases is to induce sweating and promote bowel movements. Since the cause of the disease is heat in the Liver, promoting sweating and bowel movements to eliminate dryness can cure the disease. Regardless of where the sweating occurs, be it on the forehead, eyebrows, or cheeks, as long as the sweat beads are large and disappear after a while, it is a refreshing sweat that indicates strong righteous *qi* and weak pathogenic *qi*. If the sweat beads are small and disappear quickly, it indicates weakness in the righteous *qi* and a strong pathogenic *qi*.

The pathology and pharmacology of *Tae-eumins* are incomplete and additional research is needed in the future.

4) *Soeumin*

Soeumins are healthy as long as their digestion is sound. Those who have dark facial expressions because of the indigestion, epigastric pain and fullness they constantly feel are typically *Soeumins*. Their food consumption is relatively small and they can develop diarrhea easily if they eat cold foods such as ice cream or if they drink cold beer. This is not due to problems in the intestine but rather due to the inability of the stomach to withstand the cold. A *Soeumin's* typical disease involves problems with the digestive system.

Since *Soeumins* are not obese and have cold bodies, they

should not sweat in great amounts. If they are sweating profusely, it indicates that they have developed an illness. If they sweat profusely because of over-exercising, their vitality will lessen and their bodies will become even colder so that they can easily develop an illness.

Soeumins have a weak Spleen and Stomach and this causes many diseases. Although they may fall prey to another disease, as long as there is no problem in the Spleen and Stomach, the illness is not of great concern. Regardless of the type of disease a *Soeumin* has, as long as he or she does not have much sweating and can drink water easily, it is not a serious disease. There are two auspicious signs in *Soeumin* diseases. One is sweating on DU-26 (in the philtrum) and the other is their ability to drink water. If a *Soeumin* can drink the water easily, there is sufficient *yang* energy in the Spleen and so the disease can be easily cured.

There are two urgent symptoms in *Soeumin's* disease. One is fever with profuse sweating and the other is diarrhea that is like clear water. Diarrhea in *Soeumins* must be taken seriously. Even if there are only two to three occurrences of diarrhea in a month, it must not be taken lightly. If there are four to five bouts of diarrhea in one day or if they have diarrhea for three days in a row, it indicates a serious problem. Three to four bowel movements of dry stool, even though there is no diarrhea, also indicate a serious problem.

If there is a throat problem in a *Soeumin*, even though it may be serious, it is not of great concern for it can be easily treated. Nevertheless, it still requires appropriate treatment.

The physiology and pathology of *Soeumins* are the most well known, and there are a great number of effective treatment formulas. Thus they are the easiest to treat among the four constitutions.

4. Herbal Medicines and Tonics

The treatment methods for various illnesses in SCM differ considerably from those of Traditional Chinese Medicine (Syndrome Medicine). We can follow the progression of Traditional Chinese Medicine through the many medical books written on the subject. These include, *Ben Cao* (*Shen Nung's* Herbal), written by the legendary emperor *Shen Nung* (*circa* 2800 BC), the *Nei Jing* (Inner Classic), written by the legendary Yellow Emperor (circa 2700 BC), *Shang Han Lun* (Theory of Febrile Disease Induced by Cold), written by Zhang Zhong Jing (142-220 AD) and *Huo Ren Shu* (Book for Saving Life), written by Zhu Gong (circa 11th-12th century AD). In Korea, a comprehensive description of past studies of Chinese medicine was compiled in the book, *Precious Mirror of Eastern Medicine* written by Huh Jun (1546-1615 AD).

The theories of disease syndromes and their therapeutic measures that Dr. Lee Je-ma presents in SCM do, however, bear certain resemblance to those of Traditional Chinese Medicine indicating that the constitutional theory succeeds the conventional eastern medical theory. It can, therefore supplement the weaknesses of the traditional medical view from a constitutional perspective. Nevertheless, there are fundamental differences between SCM's viewpoint of disease syndromes and treatment methods and that of Traditional Chinese Medicine, which utilizes the principle of tonifying deficiency and sedating excess. In particular, herbs are used according to each constitution. Herbs that are not appropriate for a constitution are not used in the herbal prescriptions for that constitution.

Dr. Lee Je-ma differentiated herbs that are appropriate and inappropriate for the individual constitutions according to their therapeutic nature. In addition, he classified formulas for each constitution from the books written by the famous doctors of the Song (960-1279 AD), Yuan (1279-1368 AD) and Ming (1368-1644 AD) dynasties. He also saw a need for additional formulas because the ones in existence were insufficient to treat conditions for various constitutions.

Dr. Lee Je-ma believed that the pathological syndromes and pharmacology for *Soeumins* were almost completely determined, but the syndromes and pharmacology for *Soyangins*, *Tae-eumins* and *Taeyangins* were not clearly distinguished in a descending order. In particular, there is almost no understanding of the pathological syndromes and pharmacology of *Taeyangins*.

Since there are beneficial and harmful herbs for each constitution, improper use of tonics, such as ginseng and deer horn, can result in no effect or, in extreme cases, greatly worsen a condition. In short, tonics that seem beneficial for everyone must be used according to individual constitutions or adverse reactions may occur.

The treatment of *Taeyangin* disorders focuses on nourishing the *yin* by sedating the *yang*, as *Taeyangins* have excess amounts of *yang* and a shortage of *yin*. Again, *Taeyangins* appear weak when standing because of their weak waist and legs. Herbs such as acanthopanax and pine nodes are used for diseases in the lower body. The typical diseases of *Taeyangins* include *yul-gyuk* (dysphagia), *ban-wyi* (vomiting) and *hae-yuk* (lower body weakness). For these problems, herbs and foods such as Chinese quince, grape roots, actinidia fruit (Asian kiwi), clams, Prussian carp, and water shield plants are used. Since *Taeyangins* have strong Lungs and a weak Liver, vegetables, fruits and shellfish are used to strengthen the Liver. Tonics for *Taeyangins* include acanthopanax, Chinese quince, actinidia fruit (Asian kiwi), pine needles and Prussian carp.

Soyangins also have plenty of *yang* and insufficient *yin*, so their treatment focuses on sedating the *yang* and tonifying *yin*. *Soyangins* have a strong Spleen and weak Kidneys, so herbs that strengthen the energy of the Kidneys are used. These include cooked rehmannia, cornus fruit, poria, anemarrhena, alismatis, moutan bark, phellodendron, trichosanthis seed, notopterygium, sileris, coptis, polyporus, raw rehmannia, and gypsum. Inappropriate foods and herbs such as chicken (can create a skin rash due to heat-toxins), aconite, ginseng (can cause a fever and other toxic reactions), gleditsia (can cause vomiting), and aquilaria (can cause thirst) are eliminated from the herbal prescriptions. Tonics for *Soyangins* include cooked and raw rehmannia, cornus fruit, lycium fruit, and ganoderma.

It is very important for *Tae-eumins* to urinate and move their bowels regularly as the nature of their blood is turbid and the nature of their energy is stagnant. Since *Tae-eumins* have a strong Liver and weak Lungs, their Lungs need to be strengthened. Herbs that are beneficial for them include ophiopogon, schizandra, wild yam, platycodon, cow gallstone, scutellaria, morus bark, apricot seed, ephedra, Job's tears, chestnut, bear gall bladder, and polygala. The herbs that should not be used for *Tae-eumins* include kansui root (can create a stifling sensation in the chest), cinnamon twig (can cause hives), cinnabar (can cause thirst), gypsum (can cause coldness in the extremities), bupleurum (can cause continuous perspiration) and phellodendron (can cause urinary obstruction). Tonics for *Tae-eumins* include deer horn, bear gall bladder, schizandra, ophiopogon, and kudzu.

For *Soeumins*, the treatment principle is to warm up and strengthen the blood and *qi*, because their blood and *qi* are weak and stagnant. They have strong Kidneys and a weak Spleen. Herbs that strengthen the Spleen include ginseng, white atractylodes, licorice, Chinese angelica, ligusticum, cinnamon bark, tangerine peel, peony, aconite, saussurea, cloves, and cyperus. Herbs and foods that are contraindicated for *Soeumins* include kudzu (can cause hiccups), kansui root (can cause thirst and diarrhea), buckwheat (can cause edema), rhubarb (can cause diarrhea), cinnabar (can cause *qi* rebellion leading to cold limbs), pear (can cause hiccups), ephedra (can cause thirst, excess sweating and chills), gypsum (can cause excessive phlegm and diarrhea), quisqualis (can cause hiccups), beef (can cause diarrhea), bupleurum (can increase the amount of perspiration), pork (can cause indigestion and fainting), phellodendron (can cause nausea), and coptis (can cause headaches). Tonics for *Soeumins* include ginseng, astragalus, aconite, cinnamon twig, and Chinese angelica.

Most people think that they must take drugs when afflicted with a disease. Even though they are advised to emphasize the importance of cultivating their minds as well as making dietary and lifestyle changes, they do not readily approve or accept these notions. They look forward to eliminating their trouble only by the virtue of several packs of herbal medicine.

From the viewpoint of SCM, such concepts are inappropriate. Even if a treatment is successful at eliminating one disease, unless patients make lifestyle changes and control their emotions, sooner or later, they will be susceptible to other diseases. Moreover, without changes in mental attitudes, diet and lifestyle, longevity is not a reality. Ultimately no treatment will be complete without these changes.

Fundamentally, SCM differentiates constitutional syndromes from diseases. Therefore, it is an important principle in SCM to not use herbs for syndromes that are not diseases, and to not use strong herbs for mild diseases. Health should be acquired with ordinary health cultivation methods and herbs should not be used indiscriminately.

5. Preserving Health through the Control of Emotions

In ancient times medical doctors believed that diseases were caused either by foods and drinks that injured the Spleen and Stomach or by an invasion of external pathogens such as wind, coldness, summer heat and dampness. They did not consider that imbalances in emotions such as love, hatred, desire, joy, anger, sorrow and pleasure could cause diseases.

SCM, too, considers the external pathogens as causative factors in diseases. However, SCM believes that it is a mistake to take account of only the external factors as causes of diseases. The reason for this is that under the same climatic and dietary conditions, some people are afflicted with a disease while others are not. Thus it is wrong to believe that only the external factors cause diseases. Let's look at people's diets as an example. Cold foods and drinks can cause indigestion in people who have constitutionally weak and cold Stomachs (i.e. *Soeumin*), but for people who have constitutionally strong Stomachs (i.e. *Soyangin*), they do not cause any problems.

SCM does not believe that a weak Spleen and Stomach, or a weak circulatory or respiratory system indicates only disorders in the anatomical organs. These weaknesses have an intimate relationship with the organs of the Four Burners, which are the Lungs, Spleen, Liver and Kidneys, as well as, the four emotions of sorrow, anger, joy, and pleasure. The strengths and weaknesses of the internal organs are dependent upon the appropriateness or excesses of the four emotions. Inversely, excesses of the four emotions can injure the internal organs.

Therefore, when it comes to curing diseases of the internal organs, it is insufficient to control only the energies of the organs. One's nature and emotions need to be regulated as well. SCM states that one should control one's mind in order to cure a disease. Thus, regulating one's nature and emotions is the best way to prevent or to cure a disease.

Taeyangins should be cautious about their anger and sorrow. When *Taeyangins* get angry, the emotion does not amplify slowly. Rather it explodes abruptly and then suddenly settles down. Their expression of anger can be described more precisely as a rage or fury, but again it does not last long. This sudden burst and settling of anger injures the Liver. For this reason, *Taeyangins* are cautioned to be wary of their anger. Those *Taeyangins* who feel a surge of anger should practice breathing exercises. If they cultivate this habit, they can prevent the outburst of anger from shooting upward toward the back of the head. They can also quickly settle down as they realize the trivialities of the situation.

Additionally, *Taeyangins* should not get overly emotional over sad events. They should rather feel sorrow and then forget it in the same way they inherently encounter anger. If *Taeyangins* hold tightly onto the person or event that made them sad, they can injure their internal organs and their anger will amplify.

If *Taeyangins* control their explosive anger and deep sorrow, their internal organs will be strengthened and good health will result. Otherwise, abrupt anger and deep sorrow will combine together and ascend upward to cause diseases.

In contrast to *Taeyangins*, *Soyangins* have expressive sorrow and deeply held anger. When *Soyangins* encounter a saddening event, they react in an extremely emotional manner. We can say that the sorrow wells up or that *Soyangins* fill up with sorrow. To the extent that they get sad easily, the sadness also quickly fades. This abrupt onset and settling of sorrow injures the Kidneys.

Soyangins should not become overly emotional concerning anger causing events. They should rather quickly feel the anger and then forget about it just as they react to a sad event. *Soyangins* have a tendency to bury the memories of a person or even that made them angry. It would be better for them to express their anger and keep sorrow inside. If they bury anger in their memories, not only will their internal organs be damaged, but also their sorrow will amplify.

Tae-eumins experience pleasure easily, but the sensation lasts only a very short time. Since pleasure is easily stirred up for them, they frequently laugh loudly, but soon become indifferent. This action injures the Lungs. It is, therefore, advisable for them to develop habits of staying calm by exercising self-control in their dignified and reserved physical appearance, even though they feel pleasure.

For *Tae-eumins,* pleasure is easily expressed and dissolved, whereas the emotion of joy is held within. It is beneficial for *Tae-eumins* to quickly express and release joy. If *Tae-eumins* hold onto the feeling of joy, not only will they damage their internal organs, but also pleasure will be felt even more easily.

For *Soeumins*, the feeling of joy is expressed quickly while pleasure is kept in their hearts. This joy, which can be described as the flowing tide, quickly surges and ebbs. This rapid and frequent occurrence of joy and excitement will lead to the injury of the Spleen. Therefore, it is advisable for *Soeumins* to give thought to their feelings of joy and to make it a rule to distinguish whether or not a situation is actually worth being joyful over in accordance with their usual calm and settled nature.

When *Soeumins* encounter a pleasant event, they tend to keep the pleasure deeply in their hearts without immediately expressing it outwardly. *Soeumins*, however, would do better to openly react to their feelings of pleasure as they do with joy. If they keep pleasure in their hearts too deeply, not only will the internal organs be damaged, but also their feelings of joy will be elevated.

As described above, both *Taeyangins* and *Soyangins* should always be vigilant over their emotions of anger and sorrow. Even so, they must not exaggerate or disguise their feelings of joy or pleasure. False joy and pleasure not only falsely rise from the heart but will also intensify the anger and sorrow. Both *Tae-eumins* and *Soeumins* should always be cautious of pleasure and joy, but frequent occurrences of contrived sorrow or anger will only serve to bring out even more excessive pleasure and joy.

The *Doctrine of the Mean*, one of the Four Books of Confucianism, states, "To have no stirring of the emotions of joy, anger, sorrow or pleasure is the state of the equilibrium; to have these emotions well up in due proportion is the state of harmony." No one has full control of his or her emotions from birth, but they can gain control through constant vigilance and reflection over the emotions of joy, anger, sorrow and pleasure. When the mind is controlled, the disharmony of the body will automatically be regulated.

6. Enjoying Longevity by Overcoming the Vices of Temperament

We can observe a wide variety of temperamental differences in people. Some are extremely passive in all affairs while some are overly active, which at times causes problems. Some are extremely hasty in their affairs, while some are extremely slow.

People differ in their reactions to situations such as making friends, doing work, running a household, and organizing others in a wide variety of ways. Yet, because these differences are individual idiosyncrasies, they can be both positive and negative attributes. For an assertive person, his or her assertiveness can be either a strong point or a weak point. The same is true for a passive person when it comes to his or her passiveness. Problems arise when a person's tendencies are extremely one-sided. This cannot only ruin one's work but also one's health.

Taeyangins and *Soeumins* can be seen as the extreme constitutions in terms of their positiveness. *Taeyangins* are overly positive, while *Soeumins* are overly passive. *Taeyangins*' heads are filled only with ideas of success, with little thought of failure. They can provide leadership for people who may hesitate before initiating a difficult task and they do not make the foolish mistake of losing the opportunity to begin an urgent matter. At the same time they may underestimate the difficulties that lie ahead.

The decisiveness of *Taeyangins* is not an expression of assertiveness that comes from being prepared for obstacles after evaluating what is needed for any given task. Instead, it is derived from a kind of reckless courage. Thus when an unexpected situation arises, *Taeyangins* are not able to cope with it effectively. This is because they lack the essential knowledge of what the task requires and they lack flexibility in a changing situation.

Consequently, there are two conditions in which *Taeyangins* can succeed. One is that *Taeyangins* can hastily complete a task, as long as the task is below the level of their capabilities. The other is that they need to take a step back and thoroughly investigate a task before they begin. This way they will have a better understanding of what they are up against and they can prepare for any obstacles that might lie ahead.

Soeumins may be fearful of what seems very safe to

Taeyangins. *Soeumins* have a tendency to do things that stand a good chance of success and only adopt methods that are completely safe. They do not begin a task until they have a clear picture of success. Even after starting a task, they push ahead with incessant care and circumspection.

Because of their scrupulous tendencies, *Soeumins* have less of a chance of failure. They calculate every possible consequence of their actions and are very prepared before they embark on a task, thus avoiding risks. In practice, this behavior can only bring with it small successes. Moreover, *Soeumins* frequently miss opportunities or suffer losses because they over-calculate things down to the smallest detail.

Although prudence may be a positive trait, there is a proper time for everything. If *Soeumins* worry only about failure, they may not gain anything. Thus, they must not be overly prudent. If *Soeumins* get caught up on thoughts of failure, their work will suffer as will their health. They may begin to feel a heavy sensation of the head as if a rock were on it. This will eventually ruin their health.

Soyangins and *Tae-eumins* do not appear to be extreme in terms of positive and negative work habits, but when it comes to the perseverance, they show contrasting characteristics. *Soyangins* tend to be eager when starting new projects but lack the perseverance to complete them. In contrast, *Tae-eumins* are very reluctant to start new projects, but have the tenacity and perseverance to finish what they start.

Soyangins are advised to make it a rule not to start new projects unless they have the full conviction to finish the project once it is started. There may be obstacles, but they need to muster the strength to overcome them with unrelenting perseverance. Though they may be good at starting new projects, by quitting many projects before their completion they will not have much success in terms of career and business and they will also damage their health.

Tae-eumins should not be overly reluctant or fearful about starting a new project. They tend to believe that they have the knowledge necessary to succeed with their work and are able to persist. But how can they expect things to improve if they fear new things and unconditionally feel difficulty? *Tae-eumins* should consider the work they are currently involved in as about the same as the trivial work that someone else is involved in. Everything is difficult and troublesome at first but one can soon become accustomed to it.

Unlike *Soyangins* or *Tae-eumins*, neither *Taeyangins* nor *Soeumins* show outstanding features in terms of perseverance in their work. This does not indicate that they are reluctant to start or fear new work. Once they begin a project, they show persistence to some extent.

In terms of the tough and strong masculine nature versus the soft and gentle feminine nature, *Taeyangins* are in direct contrast to *Soeumins*. *Taeyangins* are overly masculine and have few feminine characteristics, while *Soeumins* are overly feminine with few masculine traits. *Yin* and *yang* need to work together in order to maintain harmony. A tilt in either direction makes completing work and maintaining health impossible.

While exhibiting masculine traits may be suitable for *Taeyangins* regardless of their sex, there may be occasions better suited for feminine attributes. For *Soeumins*, femininity may be suitable in some situations, but depending on the circumstances, masculine characteristics may be more fitting.

Since *Soyangins* and *Tae-eumins* have both masculine and feminine characteristics to a certain degree, they are not present in an extreme of either. The difference between the two is that *Soyangins* emphasize external achievements while *Tae-eumins* focus on their inner, more domestic affairs.

Soyangins tend to have more enthusiasm for the affairs of others than for their personal dealings. They enjoy fame and recognition more than practical matters, and show a greater concern over community affairs than they do about their domestic lives. In contrast, *Tae-eumins* are overly focused on practical matters, caring only for their affairs without concern for moral obligations or reputations, making them look very greedy.

Taeyangins and *Soeumins* are unremarkable when it comes

to this issue. They both have a certain amount of interest in their personal lives and do not neglect the concerns of others.

Each constitution has its own mental tilt or inclination that can function as either a characteristic strength or can ruin the work in which each constitution is engaged. Furthermore, these dispositions can cause mental weaknesses. If people can learn to control their mental weaknesses, they can maintain their health and achieve longevity. Otherwise if their imbalance becomes greater, it will damage their health and shorten their life span.

Taeyangins express the masculine characteristic of moving blindly forward. They constantly feel a mental urgency. If they can control this urgency and calm down by adopting the attitude of "taking one step back," they can achieve longevity.

Soyangins lack perseverance and give up easily. They also show little concern for their own well-being. Due to these traits, they frequently suffer from anxiety. Thus, *Soyangins* need to pay more attention to their internal affairs. This way they can calm their anxiety and achieve longevity.

Tae-eumins hold a lot of fear around starting new projects and have a tendency to avoid working in the outside world. If they can observe the outside world with a more positive attitude, they can settle their fearful minds and achieve longevity.

Soeumins have nervous minds. They have a great deal of anxiety over what may go wrong, so they prefer to stay put. If they can take one step forward and settle their nervous minds, they can achieve longevity.

7. Appropriate Exercises

Nowadays people show unprecedented interest in health, perhaps due to the worsening of pollution and the increase in modern diseases. These concerns about health have brought prosperity to the health industries so that the fierce competition among them has become an object of public concern. We can also feel the ever-increasing concerns about pure water as people crowd around every spring well. The number of joggers in the early morning hours has also increased. Everyone is more or less practicing a method of the health cultivation according to his or her own opinions.

Have you ever consulted with people around you in order to select a suitable exercise regime? If you have, you might have been surprised to hear so many different opinions.

Some people insist on weight training. They say that a true exercise ought to involve lifting a barbell and sweating heavily. They even reason that only through such exercise, can all of the toxins in the body be eliminated.

Others speak highly of swimming. They say that swimming involves the entire body, thus providing a high intensity exercise in a short period of time. In addition it is thought to be safer than exercises performed outside of the water because there is less shock to the body's systems.

Still others regard jogging as the best exercise. They insist that humans ran for survival in primitive times and that the human body is structured to run, but due to the advent of the automobile, bodily imbalances arose.

These might be some of the moderate examples of exercise regimes. In contrast, there are some people who insist that exercise is useless. They state that there has been no remarkable evidence showing the improvement of health, and in their personal experience, exercising in the morning only reduces their appetite and makes them feel tired the whole day.

Listening to such a variety of advice can only cause confusion and difficulty in making a proper decision. Whose doctrine is right? In response, exercising is good for one's health. However, specific types of exercises are better suited for different constitutions. There is no one health cultivating method that is applicable for everyone. Each person should choose an exercise that matches his or her own physical features.

Tae-eumins should select a high-intensity exercise. They need to consume and eliminate what they voraciously eat through dynamic activities. Because *Tae-eumins* tend to pay attention not only to their own personal matters but also to their physical bodies, they have excessive greed for food, which leads to the danger of becoming obese. Their obesity can be prevented through profuse sweating by doing sufficient exercises. It is a sign of health when *Tae-eumins* sweat profusely in their daily lives and it would be beneficial to their health if they could exercise regularly to induce sweating.

It is recommended, therefore, to practice a heavy intensity exercise such as weight training or jogging for an extended time at a high speed to get a sufficient amount of exercise.

On the contrary, *Soeumins* should be careful not to choose highly intense exercises. No matter what exercise is chosen, it will not improve their health if they do it to exhaustion. The people who stated that exercise is useless since exercising lowered their appetite and made them tired were most likely *Soeumins* who exercised beyond their capabilities.

Soeumins are cautioned not to overwork themselves into exhaustion because they have constitutional weakness in their vital energy. Hence, it would be better to consider the state of their physical conditions and select exercises that do not require much energy. It is important for *Soeumins* to think of performing exercises that cover the entire body while maintaining a moderate amount of muscle tension, and developing their flexibility, rather than developing a steel-like body and big muscles through an exercise such as weight training. Exercises like calisthenics and jogging which do not overburden their bodies are recommended, as well as, quick and high intensity exercise such as tennis for a short time on regular basis. Even if it is not an exercise, the health cultivating activities that require much consumption of body energy, for example, a sauna, are likely to be only harmful for *Soeumins*.

The exercise intensity for both *Taeyangins* and *Soyangins* lie in the middle range. That is, though they are not so weak in physical strength as *Soeumins*, they need not sweat heavily every time like *Tae-eumins*.

So far we have observed the facets of stamina in each

constitution, but there are things to be considered in terms of personalities and temperaments. *Tae-eumins* do not have a strong competitive spirit and so while they may enjoy the competition itself, they do not have a strong attachment to victory. They do not have personalities that enjoy defeating the competition. Though they are not very quick, they have a great deal of energy and physical strength. In comparison, *Soyangins* have less endurance and less patience than *Tae-eumins*, but have the advantage that bravery affords them, and are quick and highly competitive.

Thus, it can be said that *Tae-eumins* would do well in sports such as wrestling or weight lifting, while *Soyangins* are well suited for sports such as boxing, table tennis, or track and field. SCM, however, is unconcerned with sports aptitude because different sports involve different and complex abilities. It is unreasonable to discern sports aptitude by constitution alone. For SCM the interest lies in determining what methods should be used to increase a person's physical and mental health.

From the perspective of SCM, strength implies a one-sided inclination, which also brings about weakness. Hence if you exercise only your strength, your weakness will be more pronounced and that will result in harm. Performing exercises or sports that can strengthen and supplement your weak areas will help the body maintain balance.

Tae-eumins should focus on sweating through heavy exercises such as wrestling or weight lifting, but at times it is necessary to perform exercises that require agility and quickness to supplement their weaknesses. For *Soyangins*, the exercises or sports that require their brave and quick nature are best, but at times they should perform exercises that develop endurance and muscle strength.

Taeyangins' active and aggressive natures make them suitable for competitive sports. When participating in team sports such as a basketball or soccer, *Taeyangins* frequently play the forward positions, as they are skilled at moving forward without retreating. In contrast, *Soeumins* dislike intensely competitive sports, and usually play defensive positions in team sports. Therefore, to overcome their physical and temperamental weaknesses, it is advisable for *Taeyangins* and *Soeumins* to switch positions sometimes.

In terms of bodily shape, *Taeyangins* and *Soyangins*, whose upper bodies are more developed than the lower bodies, need to choose exercises that help develop their lower bodies. On the other hand, *Tae-eumins* and *Soeumins* have relatively more developed lower bodies but have weak upper bodies and so need to perform exercises that can strengthen their upper bodies.

8. Talents, Aptitudes, and the Selection of a Profession

The traditional saying, "If he is a man, he should never refuse to drink a gallon of wine and should be able to lift a sack of rice without effort," seems to have little truth these days. The thought that masculinity is a symbol of courage and femininity the emblem of beauty and delicateness seems out of date.

When farming, fishing, and carpentry were the most popular professions, the symbol of manliness was muscle power. Today, when work consists of sitting at a desk with a computer, the characteristic images of manliness seem less valuable than in previous times. Because not all men have been accustomed to doing hard labor and farm work since childhood, despite physiological differences, not all men are strong with solid muscles.

As a result, the differences between the sexes have to be re-examined. The occupational distinctions between men and women have almost completely vanished. There are no longer jobs that are designated only for women or men. People are now crossing over to the previously forbidden work zones of the opposite sex.

Though there are personality differences between the sexes,

it is more important to consider the constitutional features of the sexes. This makes it possible for a man to be feminine and a woman to be masculine. It is not advisable for a feminine man, who is more suited to helping his spouse undertake work outside the home, to go out and embark on a new business venture. Ultimately, he would give up on the business because he would say that the business is not for him. In contrast, if a man confines his spouse to the home when she wants to pursue a business outside the home, her discontent may find its way into a conflict that may eventually lead to a domestic breakup.

Long ago, a citizen's profession was limited to four types: scholar, farmer, artisan, and tradesman. Today's occupational variety affords us many more options and does not limit us to only four categories of work. This variety forces people to pay great attention to their own aptitudes.

There are many people who do not feel satisfied with their current occupation. One's job should not simply be a means of earning a living. One's work should be something from which satisfaction and joy can be derived. For people whose occupations do not allow them to use their abilities or do not match their personality, the work itself can become a source of great pain. These people are fully prepared to throw away their jobs as soon as they find another means to support themselves.

What kind of a job is right for me? Naturally, the job that matches one's character and preference will bring about the most joy. Furthermore, if it is the job that allows one to display one's talents, it will bring a feeling of achievement so that work is enjoyable.

With regard to occupation, *Taeyangins*' strengths lie in their ability to communicate and take action without a hitch. No matter how trivial, they face challenges without hesitation and take clear, quick action. They are not insecure around strangers and can talk to them with ease. Because of these character traits, they have advantages when making new clients in sales or engaging in a trade or business. In a corporate business, they are well suited for the operational department. They are ideal leaders in making initial business connections for overseas operations development. They also do well in public relations.

Taeyangins are decisive and active, so they have a talent for succeeding in difficult and unknown fields. Since they associate well with people and have no fear undertaking a new business, they have the advantage in entrepreneurship and have an innate talent for business.

In terms of weaknesses in their character traits, *Taeyangins* may not be good at talking people into following them or at letting them participate in their work. They are usually not careful in their planning, are self-righteous, and have an especially rough temperament that lacks consideration for others. So, if *Taeyangins* want to succeed, they should cultivate the ability to be considerate of others by empathizing with others, or they should learn to employ people who have this ability.

Taeyangins have a talent for distinguishing a good person from a bad one, but they cannot readily distinguish a person's abilities. Without any specific standards, *Taeyangins* will employ a person of their liking, mistaking their personal feelings for ability, and they will expect a high degree of competency, while those who are not of their liking are considered untalented. Therefore, they cannot gather people of diverse talents and abilities. *Taeyangins*' ease in making acquaintances can, at most, increase their social enjoyment and make them a lot of friends. It is useless, however, in planning and carrying out a project. Furthermore, if the work turns out to be a failure, they will blame others and hold a grudge, so that people will eventually leave.

Soyangins have a warrior-like spirit and are tolerant rather than narrow-minded. They seem trustworthy in whatever is entrusted to them. They do not shirk from their duties because of self-interest and they value honor. Generally speaking, if they were placed in the auditing department of a business, they would make strict inspectors. If they were in charge of collections and disbursements, the possibility of financial accidents would be minimized. Furthermore, *Soyangins* are so diligent and honest that they often receive praise from their supervisors.

Soyangins emphasize honor more than personal profit, and value other peoples' businesses more than their own. Thus it is difficult to see them having an outstanding talent for business. However, they demonstrate fairness and reliability, and so there are many fields in which *Soyangins* can exhibit their true value, such as education or financial matters.

Soyangins lack perseverance and thus tend to give up easily when faced with difficulties. Thus, it would be safer for them to devote themselves to routine work in a stable business environment. If they want to succeed in an independent business, they need to cultivate perseverance or hire people that will constantly encourage them in difficult times.

Tae-eumins excel at maintaining their work and are persistent. But they are slow and give the impression of being clumsy. People with such a nature are appropriate for the general affairs department. Since there is a certain pattern to work in the general affairs department, there are not many unfamiliar tasks that can trouble *Tae-eumins*. In addition, the work usually involves simple, monotonous and long tasks that will quickly discourage the other constitutions, but *Tae-eumins* will not have an aversion to these tasks.

Tae-eumins would not abandon work that others view as having a small possibility of success. Moreover, once they have undertaken the work, they learn step by step to gain full knowledge of it. Thus, they have a talent for business. Since *Tae-eumins* are not progressive (*yin* type), they may not be good at venture businesses. They do, however, have a talent for common businesses such as restaurants, clothing stores, or food markets. Even though they may fail in such businesses once or twice, they do have the potential to succeed in them.

Tae-eumins are not diligent and quick in nature, so it is not advisable for them to start in an ever-changing business, such as in the information or telecommunications fields where swift responses are required. If they want to succeed in such fields, it would be better to employ people who are swift in practical tasks. It would be more suitable for *Tae-eumins* to stay back and manage these types of businesses.

Tae-eumins are very practical, but are not the type to consider the concerns of others. They clearly define their boundaries in terms of separating their own work with the work of others. Thus they look overly selfish, but have the merit of taking full responsibility for their work.

Soeumins have the advantage of being prudent and calm. They do not act thoughtlessly even in hopeless situations. They will never take action until they have a clear picture of the result. Because *Soeumins* take others into consideration, they have the gift of persuasion and can easily convince others to participate in their work. Unlike *Taeyangins*, *Soeumins* know how to distinguish between people with or without ability so that they know how to gather the right people for the job.

With such merits, *Soeumins* are suitable for a planning or a personnel department in a company. They will be good at preparing the necessary materials for beginning a new project, placing people in the proper jobs, and preparing for expected difficulties as well as balancing income and expenses. Because of their overly passive nature, they are not well suited for finalizing the project itself but rather for drafting the project or calculating and planning other complex matters that are involved.

Soeumins are not the type to throw away their current stable job and jump into a business venture. If they sufficiently investigate the venture before they begin, they will rarely fail. However, since they avoid risks, they are likely to gain only a small profit. *Soeumins* may not be destined to gaining a large profit, but since they do have the talent for gathering people of ability, if they can properly utilize this talent, they can supplement their weaknesses.

9. Selecting a Partner

To this day in Korea, there are many people who look to fortune-tellers to predict marital harmony before a marriage. Foretelling marital harmony first involves reading the Four

Pillars (birth year, month, day, and time according to the Chinese calendar) of both the bride and the groom. Then, in accordance with the Five Element Theory, a prediction is made about the future of the couple if they get married.

In the past, couples who planned to be married broke the engagement when the reading gave them a bad omen. Once a couple whose reading predicted marital harmony were married, divorce was a rare occurrence. Nowadays, while most people regard the reading of marital harmony to be a superstition, separation and divorce are common occurrences. Is it because people in the past were wiser, or are people nowadays thoughtless?

It is said that conflicting personalities is the primary reason for divorce today. When the divorcing couple loved each other, however, they must have thought they were well matched. Did love make the couple blind to their conflicting personalities or was the thing that initially drew them to the other person simply financial or educational background?

There is no relationship between the Four Pillars and SCM, but since the most common reason for divorce is said to be due to personality differences, let's look into matching personalities according to SCM.

The first question that comes to mind is whether it is advantageous for a couple to be of the same constitution. If they are of the same constitution, they will have the advantage of understanding each other well and being able to predict their partner's next course of action. It has been said that a spouse is a lost soul mate and for this reason it may not be advantageous for both persons in a relationship to be of the same constitution. In order to be attracted to one another and to grow as a couple, each partner should have different facets to their character traits. This way they can supplement each other's weaknesses.

If a couple tries only to move forward in their relationship and does not move back or if they frequently want to embark on new undertakings, there will be troubles. The former may be the case of a *Taeyangin* couple and the latter that of a *Soyangin* couple. The former couple will frequently clash because they each want to move in different directions in terms of their relationship. The latter will always taste the bitterness of failure due to making hasty decisions without preparation.

Since the number of *Taeyangins* is very small, it is very rare for two *Taeyangins* to become a couple. In a *Taeyangin* couple, if one spouse overwhelms the other, then the differing opinions will converge into one direction securing peace in the home. If this does not occur, every day will bring about some sort of conflict in this relationship. *Taeyangin* couples need to learn to make mutual concessions and to stop blaming one another.

A *Soyangin* couple will be impatient and imprudent. They will tend to make a lot of mistakes in everything they do and will quarrel frequently. Moreover, additional family problems will arise since they tend to focus more on outside affairs and neglect their domestic affairs. In this relationship, however the quarrels do not last long and both partners are diligent so that they can live a happy and joyful life together. If a *Soyangin* couple wants to live in harmony, at least one spouse must cultivate a more serious attitude.

A *Tae-eumin* couple seems more like two friends than a pair of lovers. They are both serious and patient. They do not meddle in the affairs of their partner nor do they like people to interfere in their affairs. Thus they do not often clash with one another. Each spouse in this relationship takes responsibility for him or herself, which means that they can run household business smoothly. When they do experience conflict, however, it can often proliferate due to their stubbornness. Since *Tae-eumins* do not take meticulous care of each other, they can easily begin to feel indifferent toward one another. In order for a *Tae-eumin* couple to have a harmonious married life, each spouse must learn to express his or her interest in their partner by celebrating their anniversary or remembering the birthday of their partner and having a surprise party or going out to a show.

A *Soeumin* couple appears to have no particular problems in their married life. *Soeumins* are tactful and considerate of each other's feelings, so as long as the initial affection remains, it is rare for them to have much conflict. Because they can hold onto an emotional hurt over a trivial matter for a long time, a *Soeumin* couple must learn to be indifferent to these hurts.

Couples of the same constitution can easily adjust their diets to be in tune with one another, which is beneficial to their health. The list of foods that can be enjoyed by a couple of two different constitutions, however, may be in conflict.

Now, let's consider the cases of couples with different constitutions since these cases tend to be more common.

A *Tae-eumin-Soeumin* couple may give off an image of a taciturn husband with a tender wife or a meticulous husband with a clumsy wife. Because they are both *yin* constitutions, they are not progressive. A *Soeumin* is likely to complain about a *Tae-eumin*'s lack of appeal, and the *Tae-eumin* is likely to blame his or her partner for being too inquisitive.

Although *Tae-eumins* and *Soyangins* are very different in character, as a couple their differences may actually serve to supplement each other's weaknesses. *Soyangins* will create a fun and happy family with their charm, which balances the bluntness, tactlessness, and selfish behaviors of *Tae-eumins*. A *Tae-eumin* can prevent a *Soyangin* from making mistakes due to their frivolous and hasty nature. *Soyangins* think much of the things in the outside world, while the *Tae-eumins* care for domestic affairs. These differences will help to bring fruitfulness both inside and outside of the relationship. When the conflicting personalities clash to create domestic discord, it can lead to irreversible differences due to mutual misunderstandings. Often what seems like an attractive quality in a partner when there is affection becomes a flaw when the love cools down? As long as this is kept in mind, the *Tae-eumin-Soyangin* couple will be able to lead a harmonious married life.

Since there are also personality differences in a *Soyangin-Soeumin* couple, this relationship can become mutually complementary. A *Soeumin* can understand the extroverted tendency of a *Soyangin* to a certain degree and a *Soyangin* would not be concerned with the overly introverted tendency of a *Soeumin*. If a *Soyangin* always tries to embark on a new undertaking without finishing them, then a *Soeumin* will become annoyed. Also, if a *Soeumin* is always reluctant or backs down from beginning new work due to his or her worries over trivial things, then a *Soyangin* will begin to feel stifled.

This situation would not cause any trouble for *Tae-eumins* because they are also slow in starting new work. To remedy these problems, *Soeumins* should sometimes trust the decisions of *Soyangins*, and *Soyangins* should always keep in mind not to start new projects beyond their abilities and if they do, the projects should be completed. In this way they will be able to prevent conflicts in their relationship.

When *Taeyangins* are married to a spouse of a different constitution, they need to eliminate their self-righteous attitudes and take time to listen to their spouse. This is the art of maintaining a harmonious marriage.

Part II

Understanding Sasang Constitutional Medicine

Chapter 4
Understanding Sasang Constitutional Medicine

The first three chapters of this book were written for the general public in an attempt to give the readers a basic understanding of the complex principles of SCM and to allow them to apply the principles to their daily lives. The information in the first three chapters is sufficient for those who are not practicing SCM in the medical field. That being said, the general public holds some misunderstandings about SCM. The purpose of this chapter is to explain the most fundamental principles of SCM as well as to clear up the misunderstood aspects of SCM.

Those who do not have a background in Eastern medicine might feel intimidated by the information in this chapter, but those who are thoroughly acquainted with the information in the first three chapters should be able to understand it to some extent. It is, therefore, recommended that one reread the first three chapters after reading this chapter.

1. What Is Constitutional Medicine?

For a long time, both eastern and western medical practitioners have been using standardized methods in their examinations of people for diseases, implying a neglect of individual differences based on each constitution. This is not only a significant obstacle in the prevention and effective treatment of disease, but also a cause for many other problems, such as misdiagnosis or unforeseen side effects from drugs.

A patient's constitution will determine the inherent weakness of internal organs, the progression of a disease, and reactions to medications. Keeping this in mind, methods of health cultivation, treatment protocols and proper medicinal treatments for various diseases should vary according to each constitution. This is why constitutional medicine is so significant.

SCM is a new and unique constitutional medicine that was created at the end of the 19th century by Dr. Lee Je-ma. He wrote two books called *Longevity and Life Preservation in Eastern Medicine* (*Dong-ui susebowon*) and *Manuscript of Science* (*Gyeokchigo*). In his books, he classified constitutional types of human beings into *Taeyangin, Tae-eumin, Soyangin,* and *Soeumin* and researched physiology, pathology, treatment methods and health cultivation for each constitution.

TCM originated from the *Inner Classic (Nei Jing)* and the *I Ching*, following the tradition of Huang-Lao (Yellow Emperor and Lao Tzu) Sect. In comparison, SCM is a more humanity-oriented philosophy and medicine that have its foundation in the reformed school of Confucianism, which came to the forefront of the Realistic School (Pragmatism) of thought in Korea.

Dr. Lee Je-ma distinguished each constitutional type not only from a single, limited perspective but also researched a wide variety of categories, in terms of both mind and body, which include speech, conduct and personality, physical shapes, and so forth. His research took a quantum leap from its beginning when it was essentially a study of medicine to its culmination as a profound study of humanity.

People frequently think of SCM simply as a constitutional classification method. But this is not true. SCM not only classifies constitutions, it also inquires into the inevitable cause of constitutional differences. Moreover, it discusses the health and disease of people who are born with the prenatal peculiarities of any given constitution, and the correct attitude to maintain for self-cultivation. SCM explores how people can independently govern their speech and behavior as well as their minds in order to maintain a healthy body and achieve longevity. It also allows people to live their lives in a harmonious way as true human beings. For these reasons SCM is considered not simply a medicine but also a philosophy and study of humanity.

Past attempts have been made to classify people according to a few specific constitutional types. Galen's "Constitutional Theory" and the "Theory of Five Types of Humans" in the *Inner Classic* are a few examples. Hippocrates, who is known as the father of western medicine, advocated the theory that a human body is created from the four humors of blood, phlegm, bile, and black bile.

Approximately 500 years later, Galen distinguished four human temperaments based on Hippocrates' theory and labeled them "sanguine," "phlegmatic," "choleric," and "melancholic." A sanguine temperament is said to be warmhearted, social, emotional, easily excited, and cheerful while a phlegmatic temperament is dispassionate, passive, have a great deal of patience, and are obstinate. A choleric temperament is impatient, sentimental, brave, and objective, while a melancholic temperament is patient and persistent, but gloomy with subjective and conservative tendencies. Metaphorically speaking, Galen's temperamental classifications of humanity can be thought of as the business type, the scholar type, the patriotic type, the heroic type, the religious type, the moralistic type, etc. These are hypothesis that were created prior to any anatomical or physiological research. In terms of lineage, this primitive research was later supported by work in endocrinology and neurology.

The *Inner Classic*, which is the original text of Eastern medicine, mentions the Theory of Five Body Types according to the *yin-yang* Theory and the Theory of the 25 Body Types based on the Five Element Theory. The Theory of the Five Body Types was based on the concept of a *yin-yang* Harmonized Person and four others, which are classified according to their tilt of *yin* and *yang*. They are people of *taeyang*, *tae-eum*, *soyang*, and *soeum*. The 25 body types are derived from the Five Elements (wood, fire, earth, metal, and water) and each element again is divided into five subtypes. These theories distinguished the varieties in human characteristics but it is hard to see medical value in them.

Taeyang, *tae-eum*, *soyang*, and *soeum* as mentioned in the Theory of Five Body Types are the same terms that are used in SCM; however, these two theories are completely different. The Theory of the Five Body Types in the *Inner Classic* is a classification based on the relative properties of *yin* and *yang*. In SCM, the classification is based on the *Four Principles*[7] of mind and body (internal organs). What this means is that the classification of the four constitutions is based on observations of both mind and body in order to study how the mind and body differ in each person and how they are related.

In Eastern medicine, there are two methods of treatment, one based on syndrome differentiation and the other based on constitution. Prior to the presentation of the Sasang Constitutional Theory by Dr. Lee Je-ma in 1894, syndrome differentiation was the most popular treatment method and the concept of constitution was only vaguely known.

After Dr. Lee Je-ma explained the Sasang constitutions and their physiology, pathology, treatment, and pharmacology in *Longevity and Life Preservation in Eastern Medicine*, constitutional medicine was able to fully develop for the first time.

Syndrome Medicine applies the same standards to everyone, regardless of his or her constitution. As a matter of fact, individual characteristics are ignored. The causes of disease are found in the external factors such as wind, cold, summer heat, dampness, dryness, and heat, which influence the body, while individual weaknesses and peculiarities are overlooked. In contrast, it is the view of SCM that each individual has the ability to regulate his or her own body, and that the causes of disease depend upon the individual's particular characteristics of mind and body. Thus the primary cause of disease is believed

---

7) activity, mind, body, and matter.

to come from within the individual.

Because of these different processes, treatment methods are also different. The concept of *excess* and *deficiency* is very important in Syndrome Medicine. Diseases are caused either from a deficiency of Righteous *qi* or an excess of pathogenic *qi*. The fundamental treatment involves using tonification methods for deficiencies and sedation methods for excesses.

SCM views the primary cause of disease, however, to be an imbalance in the functional strength of the internal organs, which is different for each constitution. Thus, the goal in treatment is to restore balance. When the unbalanced organs are regulated, the deficiencies and the excesses adjust automatically. Therefore, there is no significance attached to classifying treatment herbs according to their tonifying and sedating properties.

In addition, because SCM views the primary causes of disease as imbalances of mind and body, it gives no weight to treatments that solely focus on exterior causes or depend only upon herbal medicine. SCM attaches great importance to controlling various emotions such as joy, anger, sorrow, pleasure, love, hate, and desire. Because of these factors, SCM is seen as a medicine that treats diseases by recognizing the significance of the patient's state of mind and how it can adversely affect the patient's health.

2. Origin and Birth of Sasang Constitutional Medicine

People differ widely in appearance, personality, hobbies, peculiarities, habits, constitution, etc. Therefore the same disease can manifest with different symptoms in different people due to variations in constitution, personality, life styles, and interests. Thus, effective treatment for different people will most likely involve different diagnostic symptoms, methods and prescriptions.

Rather than treating a person based on the cause of the

disease and the symptoms, it is most desirable to treat an individual according to their constitutional characteristics and to plan a countermeasure by discovering the progression and prognosis of the disease that corresponds to the constitutional peculiarities.

Dr. Lee Je-ma's SCM established constitutional types by classifying similar patterns, and expanded the theory to include preventive medicine. Each of Dr. Lee Je-ma's Sasang constitutional types, which are *Taeyangin, Tae-eumin, Soyangin,* and *Soeumin,* has different characteristics and so there are different patterns of diseases and treatment methods for each type. SCM systematized not only constitutional classification, but disease patterns and corresponding prescriptions, as well.

SCM is a new and original theory developed through the analysis and research of chapter 72 of the "*lingshu*" or "Spiritual Axis" of the *Inner Classic*. Dr. Lee Je-ma studied the classifications of the five constitutions, and then added his own interpretations and revisions. He said, "I was referencing the old writings of Eastern medicine which originated over five thousand years ago, and was able to discover the physiological characteristics of the internal organs of the four constitutions by chance. The Six Channel Disease Theory (*Shang Han Lun*) of Zhang Zhong-jing came from the perspective of syndromes but Sasang Constitutional Theory is a new theory based on humans themselves." His statement clearly indicates the originality of his theory (The Theory of Six Channel Diseases classifies diseases into Three *yang* and three *yin* categories, which are *taiyang, shaoyang, yangming, taiyin, shaoyin*, and *jueyin*. These are the classifications of diseases, not of people.)

Although Dr. Lee Je-ma was a medical doctor, he was fundamentally a Confucian scholar. SCM was created from his research on Confucianism. It was not the result of research originally aimed at creating a new form of medicine. So, in its creation, SCM differs from TCM. While searching for a method of self-cultivation that adhered to the principles of Confucianism, Dr. Lee Je-ma realized that individuals differ in their mental nature. These differences have both strengths and weaknesses and require different cultivation methods. In this way people can learn to cultivate himself or herself in an appropriate manner, which will allow them to grow and to serve others. So the origin of SCM stems from the idea of cultivating one's mind and body to follow in the spirit of Confucianism.

As previously mentioned, the term "Sasang" originated from the Theory of the Five Body Types in chapter 72 of the "*Ling Shu*" of *Inner Classic*. Four of the body types are *Tae-eumin, Soeumin, Taeyangin and Soyangin*. The fifth is the *yin-yang* harmonized person, who, it is believed, does not exist because harmony of the mind and body is merely a goal that is attempted through the cultivation and regulation of an unbalanced person. The remaining concepts of SCM are not borrowed from the *Inner Classic*, rather they are derived from the Activity-Mind-Body-Matter Theory of Confucianism.

Syndrome Medicine, generally called Traditional Chinese Medicine (TCM), is based on the *yin-yang* and Five-Element Theories of Taoism. These two theories have greatly influenced eastern history as followers of these theories have made grand contributions to the development of astrology, politics, medicine, and much more.

Syndrome Medicine is based on the restraining and inciting principles, or the controlling and promoting cycles of the Five Elements. In comparison, SCM is based on the theory of the *Four Principles* and the Four Burners and, rather than being tied to Taoism, SCM has an intimate relationship with Confucianism. The social situation of the time greatly influenced its formation.

Dr. Lee Je-ma was born in 1837 and died in 1900. He introduced his theory only one hundred years ago. During his time, there was such societal abuse of the Neo-Confucianism philosophies that Dr. Lee Je-ma strongly felt it was his mission to transcend it and to create a new philosophy and a new thought. SCM and the Sasang philosophy were the outcome of this mission.

The original Confucianism is based on the teachings of Confucius and Mencius. Their theory was passed on through the Han (206 BC-220 AD) and Tang (618-907 AD) dynasties and became Neo-Confucianism in the Song dynasty (960-1279 AD). At that time, Cheng Zi (1033-1107 AD) and Zhu Xi (1130-1200 AD) used the *taichi* Diagram Theory, initially advocated by Zhou Don I (1017-1073 AD), to philosophize Confucianism. But the *taichi* Diagram Theory was originally a method to explain the evolution of the universe and was derived from Taoism, similar to the *I Ching*. It states that the *taichi* produced the Two Modes (*yin* and *yang*), and the Two Modes gave rise to Sasang[8] and the Sasang divides into the Eight Trigrams. This clearly shows that the *taichi* Diagram Theory and the *I Ching* Theory of the Huang-Lao school are one and the same.

According to Zhu Xi, all objects have their own attributes, and within each attribute are material components and the mind. The material aspect refers to an object's exterior and the mind refers to its interior. Within the mind is nature and emotion. Nature is also called *tao* Mind (True Heart/higher mind) and emotion is also called Personal Mind (Personified Heart/lower mind). The *taichi* is also referred to as the *li* (organizing principle/universal law) while *yin-yang* is referred to as the *qi* (all manifestations). According to this theory, the form and function relationship of the *li* and *qi* exists between the *taichi* and *yin-yang*. Therefore, if a certain principle exists, the phenomenon of *qi* will manifest according to that principle. It is in this way that Neo-Confucianism uses the *taichi* Diagram Theory to philosophize Confucianism and explains that all organizing principles are established in the inner nature and the *qi* of all phenomena belong to *yin* and *yang*.

For seven hundred years, from the middle of the Goryeo dynasty (918-1392 AD) when Neo-Confucianism was first transmitted to Korea, to the end of the Lee or Chosun dynasty (1392-1910 AD), Neo-Confucianism prospered. With this prosperity came the corresponding corruption. The development of Neo-Confucianism in Korea was mainly due to two philosophers, Lee Toe-gye (1501-1570 AD) and Lee Yul-gok

---

8) *taeyang, tae-eum, soyang,* and *soeum* (*taiyang, taiyin, shaoyang,* and *shaoyin).*

(1536-1584 AD). Their theories surpassed those advocated by Cheng Zi and Zhu Xi and developed into an ontological theory.

Lee Toe-gye advocated the Duality Theory of *li* and *qi* while Lee Yul-gok propagated the Unitary Theory of *li* and *qi*. Through these two philosophers, Neo-Confucianism grew in Korea. The revival of Neo-Confucianism, as represented by Lee Toe-gye and Lee Yul-gok during the middle of the Chosun dynasty, became the main cause of strife among the political factions. It also led to a situation in which Zhu Xi's Neo-Confucianism controlled all social happenings, including politics. Thus, Neo-Confucianism did not remain as a philosophical idea; instead it grew into a tool to control the government, society, and eventually the people. This phenomenon led to a connection between doctrinal factions and the authorities, similar to the current illicit connections between politics and economic factions, which inevitably led to bloody power struggles. A small number of scholars rebelled against Neo-Confucianism, which focused excessively on impractical theories that were used as tools for party factions. These men gave rise to pragmatic science.

The spirit of practical science that began to spring up in society was further developed through influences of western civilization that came through the Ching dynasty (1644-1911 AD) of China. The period in which Dr. Lee Je-ma lived was a time in which such pragmatic thought was roaring. The purpose of practical science was to overthrow the theory of Neo-Confucianism and unfold a new system of Confucianism, called Reformed Confucianism. It has been said that the Sasang philosophy, the cornerstone of Dr. Lee Je-ma's SCM, is typical of Reformed Confucianism.

3. Sasang Philosophy and Sasang Constitutional Medicine

Dr. Lee Je-ma explained his philosophy using the

transitional processes of *taichi*, *yin-yang*, and Sasang, which are the principles of the *I Ching*, and completely excluded the Five Element Theory. In contrast, Zhou Don-i's *taichi* Diagram Theory was an attempt to explain Confucian thought through the developmental process of the *I Ching*.

As previously mentioned, the *I Ching* is a Taoist theory of the Huang-Lao school. The *yin-yang* and Five-Element theory are a branch of Taoism and constitute the fundamental framework of Eastern medicine discussed in the *Inner Classic (Nei Jing)*. Eastern medicine is a Syndrome Medicine that is based on these two theories from the Huang-Lao school. These theories are the mainstream traditions of eastern philosophy that have been handed down to astrologers, politicians, doctors, etc. Traditionally those who follow the principles laid out in the *yin-yang* and Five Element Theories are called *yin-yang* Tacticians.

The word "Sasang" is from the *I Ching* and refers to *taeyang*, *soyang*, *tae-eum*, and *soeum*. These words are different from those used in Dr. Lee Je-ma's Sasang Theory. Dr. Lee Je-ma reinterpreted Sasang as "activity, mind, body, and matter." These are the Sasang of human beings.

The Sasang constitutions (*Taeyangin*, *Soyangin, Tae-eumin*, and *Soeumin*) originated from the Theory of the Five Body Types presented in the *Inner Classic (Nei Jing)*. So although Dr. Lee Je-ma created the Sasang Constitutional Theory, the term "Sasang" comes from the *I Ching*, or from the Huang-Lao school, and is an explanatory term referring to the phenomena of the variations of *yin* and *yang*. Although the terms are the same, Dr. Lee Je-ma's Sasang philosophy was organized according to the Theory of Activity, Mind, Body, and Matter. Thus it is a different perspective compared with the Sasang of the *I Ching*.

In Dr. Lee Je-ma's book *Manuscript of Science*, there is a chapter entitled, "Summary of Confucianism." This particular chapter begins with an explanation of the Theory of Activity, Mind, Body, and Matter. Viewed in this light, Dr. Lee Je-ma's original intention was to develop the Sasang philosophy rather than Sasang medicine.

In order to expand the idea of Reformed Confucianism within his philosophical system, Dr. Lee Je-ma questioned the way people lived and accomplished their goals in life following the practical ethics of Confucianism. This was not only in reference to the mind but also in reference to the body. It, therefore, developed into a question of conflict between mind and body, a conflict that could impede the cultivation of character and finally lead to serious disease. These ideas led to the formation of SCM.

Once the organic relationship between the mind and the body is understood, the purpose of medicine broadens and is no longer viewed simply as a method for treating disease. There is an indivisible relationship between the health of the body and the cultivation of the mind. SCM, therefore, is a methodology that teaches people how to live in order to attain a balance between mind and body and inversely, how to modify or transform oneself in daily life in order to cultivate character.

Indeed the Sasang medical theory arose from Sasang philosophy. SCM is not simply a medicine to treat disease but is the methodology that developed from the process of mental cultivation. This is the significance of SCM. Therefore, SCM differs greatly in origin and content from the Syndrome Medicine of the *Inner Classic (Nei Jing)*. These are the reasons to affirm SCM as Dr. Lee Je-ma's original medicine.

To reiterate, SCM is based on Confucianism rather than on the Taoism of the Huang-Lao school. Even though it is based on Confucianism, it is not associated with the Neo-Confucianism of Cheng Zi or Zhu Xi, but is a medicine that developed from Reformed Confucianism. The ultimate goal of SCM is to cultivate the mind in order to achieve the proper balance of mind and body, which will lead to good health and longevity. This is the fundamental concept of this medicine.

The two basic practices of Confucianism are self-cultivation and providing service to others. These are taught in the two books, *Doctrine of the Mean* and *Great Learning*. The methodology that teaches the ways to study these practices is described in the doctrines of Neo-Confucianism. Few can object to the ideas of self-cultivation and providing service to others. However, there are many different ways to accomplish these goals, such as those stressed by Neo-Confucianism or those mentioned in the teachings of Wang Yang Ming (1472-1528 AD). SCM is one such method and was Dr. Lee Je-ma's methodology of self-cultivation and public service.

The ideas of self-cultivation and service to others are based on Confucianism. However, during the middle and latter part of Chosun dynasty, they created social disorder and strife among the political factions because politicians were attempting to govern others without first cultivating themselves. Dr. Lee Je-ma's methodology allows people to cultivate themselves fully. This method states that, "To rectify and cultivate the mind, it is equally as important to understand others as it is to understand one's self and one's weaknesses." In this way, self-cultivation can be accomplished naturally.

Dr. Lee Je-ma began his philosophical book, *Manuscript of Science,* when he was 45 years old. Ten years later, he completed the chapter called "Summary of Confucianism" *at the age of 55.* During that time, at the age of 47, he wrote another chapter called "Self-cultivation," which is a methodology on how to know others. Neo-Confucianism holds that within each human being there exist an original nature and emotions. Emotions are considered vices or evils of the mind, but according to Dr. Lee Je-ma's "Self-cultivation" we all have a virtuous "nature" and selfish "desire."

When this is broken down into further detail, we arrive at the four virtuous natures of benevolence, righteousness, propriety, and wisdom, and the four selfish desires of rudeness, superficiality, greed and indolence. These characteristics apply to everyone. There are no exceptions. Even a sage carries both a virtuous nature and selfish desires. However, a sage will have more virtuous nature than selfish desire while ordinary people have more selfish desire than virtuous nature. People are not born with fundamentally differing natures and desires. A person can become a sage or a commoner depending on his or her developing and maturing of their character.

In the past, people thought that sages were predestined. Many Confucians, including Zhu Xi, held this belief and did not believe that a person could become a sage through his own efforts. People also believed that sages were responsible for the leadership of the commoners who were considered inferior and that the commoners had a responsibility to follow the teachings of the sages. Dr. Lee Je-ma's view was a bit more rational. He believed that all people, even Confucius and Mencius were the same but that certain people became sages as the result of their efforts. Is this not a Reformed Confucianism way of thinking?

This view holds that all people have both virtuous nature and selfish desire. So, in order to understand others and the workings of their inner minds, it is necessary to first understand people's mental desires. This can be accomplished using the standardized constitutional methodology of interpreting mental desires.

While Dr. Lee Je-ma was analyzing people's mental characteristics, he discovered that similarities could not be determined from person to person, but that there was a uniformed pattern by which people could be classified. *Yin* and *yang* constitutions are determined at birth. The *yang* constitutions are *Taeyangin* and *Soyangin*, while the *yin* constitutions are *Tae-eumin* and *Soeumin*. Although each person holds within themselves the four mental desires (rudeness, superficiality, greed and indolence), the degree to which they are expressed in each constitution is different.

Taeyangins express rudeness most easily while *Tae-eumins* express greediness and avariciousness most easily. These tendencies led to the discovery of the relationship between constitutional attributes and mental desires. Applying this relationship to daily life can enlighten us to the mentality of others as well as helping us to regulate our own minds. This implies that gaining an understanding of others will lead to self-rectification and is a means by which we can cultivate our characters.

Understanding these desires and how their expressions can be damaging to one's health will lead to a knowing of how to repress one's own selfish desires. Knowing others, meanwhile, allows one to interact with others in a harmonious way. This will eventually lead to a path of self-rectification. A constitutional theory that illustrates methods of knowing others allows for self-rectification as well. This constitutional self-rectification is SCM.

To this point SCM has been explained in a philosophical sense. Dr. Lee Je-ma's SCM should not be understood only within the narrow parameters of diseases and their treatments. SCM's methods for proper daily living are its most important attributes; however, it is important to know how to treat disease when it occurs. By healing the diseases of the body and transforming the mind, one rises to a higher level of self-cultivation. Therefore, SCM must be seen from the viewpoint of a system that manages the entire process of being; knowing how to live daily life, knowing how to treat disease, and knowing how to rise to the higher level of self-cultivation.

4. The Basic Principles of Sasang Constitutional Medicine: The Differences between the Five Elements and Four Burners

Compared to TCM, in which there are Five *zang* and Six *fu* organs, there are only Four *zang* and Four *fu* organs in SCM. The Heart is excluded from the Five *zang* organs and is considered to be the mind. The Four Burners, which are the Lungs, Spleen, Liver, and Kidneys, represent the body, while the Heart represents the mind.

The Upper, Upper-Middle, Lower-Middle, and Lower Burners are related to the four emotions: sorrow, anger, joy, and pleasure. The Upper Burner is related to sorrow, the Upper-Middle Burner is related to anger, the Lower-Middle Burner is related to joy, and the Lower Burner is related to pleasure. The emotions of anger and sorrow cause physical excitement and make one's energy rise upward. Joy and pleasure will initially create emotional excitement but will later bring a person to a relaxed state. Both joy and anger cause excitement but the type of excitement is different. Excitement from joy cools quickly and drops downward, while excitement from anger does not.

Joy and pleasure cause *qi* to drop downward while anger and sorrow cause *qi* to rise. The Lungs and Spleen hold the *qi* of anger and sorrow while the Kidneys and the Liver hold the *qi* of joy and pleasure. These emotions are connected to the ascending and descending energies of the internal organs.

There are great differences between the concept of the Five Elements from the *Inner Classic (Nei Jing)* and the Four Burners. Although the names of internal organs in the Five Element system and SCM are similar, their functions are very different.

For example, the Spleen from the *Inner Classic (Nei Jing)* is referred to as the Earth element according to the Five Element Theory. Wood promotes Fire, Fire promotes Earth and Wood controls the Earth. The Liver *qi* and the Heart *qi* assist each other and the Heart *qi* and the Spleen *qi* assist each other, but the Liver *qi* restrains the Spleen *qi*. In this way, the Wood, Fire, Earth, Metal, and Water elements of the Five Element Theory relate to one another and create the suppressing and accelerating relationships needed to maintain physical balance. If the balance is lost, disease will occur.

The medicine rooted in the *Inner Classic (Nei Jing)* is based on the idea of maintaining balance, so the concepts of excess and deficiency are important. If the *qi* is in a state of excess or deficiency, a disease is present. If the *qi* is excessive, it is called an *Excess Syndrome* and if it is deficient, it is called a *Deficient Syndrome.*

The basic idea of SCM is the constitutionally differing mind and body due to variations in the internal organs. The theory holds that individuals have a congenital difference between the sizes of the internal organs. Those who have large Lungs and a small Liver are called *Taeyangin*, while those who have a large Liver and small Lungs are called *Tae-eumin*. Those who have a large Spleen and small Kidneys are called *Soyangin* while those who have large Kidneys and a small Spleen are called *Soeumin*.

If the energy of the large organ becomes more excessive or the small organ becomes more deficient, disease can occur. Disease is more likely if the nature and emotions of sorrow, anger, joy, and pleasure are excessive or become urgent. However, this gradual or sudden change in the energy of the organs, whether excessive or deficient, will not change the constitution.

SCM excludes the Five Element Theory and establishes the Four Burner Theory. The Upper Burner relates to the Lungs, the Upper-Middle Burner relates to the Spleen, the Lower-Middle Burner relates to the Liver, and the Lower Burner relates to the Kidneys. The Four Burner Theory is not based on the generating and controlling cycles of the Five Element Theory; rather it is based on the energetic relationship between the upper and lower regions. Thus, the most significant organ relationship in SCM is the ascending and descending movement of the *qi* of the Four Burners.

Qi movement is classified into ascending and descending motions. The two ascending motions are straight up and obliquely upward, while the two descending motions are obliquely downward and straight down. The emphasis is on how the energy goes up or down. The energy of the Lungs ascends straight up while that of Spleen ascends obliquely upward. The energy of the Liver descends obliquely downward while that of the Kidneys descends straight down quickly.

The Five Element Theory uses the concept of cyclical motion (promoting, controlling, overacting, and counteracting) rather than the concept of ascending and descending motions. Therefore, although the term "Spleen" is used in both SCM and Syndrome Medicine, its meaning is different, so treatment techniques must be different. It is not wise to mix formulas from SCM with those from Syndrome Medicine.

According to Syndrome Medicine, the Spleen is situated in

the position of the Earth element. It is controlled by Liver *qi* and strengthened by Heart *qi*. But according to SCM, the Spleen is positioned in the Upper-Middle Burner, which raises *qi* obliquely upward, and is intimately related to the nature of anger and the emotion of sorrow[9)] or the nature of sorrow and the emotion of anger[10)].

Dr. Lee Je-ma was originally a Confucian scholar and not a doctor. The origin of his Sasang principles can be traced back to the *Four Principles* or the *Four Beginnings*. The *Four Principles* refer to benevolence, righteousness, propriety and wisdom as mentioned in the book *Mencius*. The *Four Principles* imply four corners or foundations. If the mind can be divided into its original nature and its inclinations or desires, the four boundaries of original nature can be seen as the *Four Principles* of benevolence, righteousness, propriety and wisdom. When viewed from this perspective, SCM originated from Confucianism and can therefore be called the Four Principle Medicine.

Dr. Lee Je-ma said in his book, *Longevity and Life Preservation in Eastern Medicine*, "the vast-flowing *qi* (moral courage devoid of any shame that is deeply rooted in morality and is exceedingly just and fair) comes from the body and the vast-flowing Principle comes from the mind." Because benevolence, righteousness, propriety and wisdom are from the body, if the *qi* of the four *zang* organs is amplified, the *vast flowing qi* issues forth. And if the desires of the mind (rudeness, superficiality, greed and indolence) are discerned, the *vast flowing Principle* issues forth.

The person that Dr. Lee Je-ma most revered was Mencius

---

9) **Soyangin:** In a *Soyangin,* the nature of anger is widely encompassing so the Qi flows into the Spleen and the Spleen Qi becomes excessive. In addition, the emotion of sorrow is quick causing the Qi to stimulate the Kidneys and the Kidney Qi to become depleted. This is why *Soyangin*'s organ formation is "a large Spleen and small Kidneys."

10) **Taeyangin**: In a *Taeyangin,* the nature of sorrow is distantly dispersed so the Qi flows into the Lungs and the Lungs Qi becomes excessive. In addition the emotion of anger is quick so the Qi stimulates the Liver, and the Liver Qi becomes depleted. This is why *Taeyangin*'s organ formation is "large Lungs and a small Liver."

because he was so effective at self-cultivation and at controlling his mind. The vast-flowing *qi* that he mentioned is the immovable mind that has been freed from all things and affairs. In order to do this, it is necessary to preserve the clarity of one's mind and cultivate one's nature. One's mind must stay vigilant at all times and one's nature must be cultivated. Then the *Four Principles* of one's nature or virtuous mind, which are benevolence, righteousness, propriety and wisdom, issue forth.

But the mind has both original nature and emotions. And within the emotions is greedy desire. If the mind does not fall prey to this greedy desire, it becomes virtuous; otherwise the mind becomes wicked. The motivation for greedy desire and eventual trouble develop during the process of hearing and seeing all matters and affairs. In other words, the mind can ultimately become wicked due to temptations and affections for brilliance or splendor, as well as, greed. Therefore it is necessary to always restrain one's mind, maintain the virtuous mind and not become careless.

The terms that appear in *Longevity and Life Preservation in Eastern Medicine*, such as "A Discourse on the Four Principles," "A Discourse on the Establishment and Supplement," as well as, benevolence, righteousness, propriety and wisdom, and sorrow, anger, joy and pleasure all originate from Mencius. It is therefore, understandable for SCM to be called the Four Principle Medicine.

Needless to say, Dr. Lee Je-ma's *Four Principles* not only include sorrow, anger, joy and pleasure, as well as, benevolence, righteousness, propriety and wisdom, but also encompasses *taeyang*, *soyang*, *tae-eum*, and *soeum*, as well as, activity, mind, body and matter. Nonetheless, the foundation of his theory is always rooted in the *Four Principles* of benevolence, righteousness, propriety and wisdom, as well as in sorrow, anger, joy and pleasure.

When SCM is discussed, most people quickly relate it to *taeyang*, *soyang*, *tae-eum*, and *soeum*. Because of this, the original spirit of the *Four Principles* is neglected and SCM is treated simply as a constitutional theory.

5. The Constitutions Do Not Change Over Time

The constitutions are congenital and do not change over time. The sizes of the organs are predetermined from the time of birth. However, the personality develops postnatally and is variable. Since the congenital nature cannot be changed, the variable factors must be regulated and well managed to maintain balance. One of the most important teachings of SCM is that in order to correct the invariable body one must control the variable mind. The bodily constitution is predetermined but control of the mind depends upon the effort of the individual. Therefore diseases of the body could also be treated through the cultivation of the mind.

Although this may sound silly, I once heard of a person that was classified as a *Soeumin* when he was young. As he got older his introverted personality disappeared and it is said that he became a *Soyangin.* Obviously this is not true since the constitution never changes. In this instance, it was not the man's body that changed but his mind.

According to TCM (Syndrome Medicine), if a person is overweight during her entire childhood but becomes very thin as she gets older, this person's constitution has changed over time. Another person may think that because he had a problem with his liver in the past but now has a severe problem in his stomach, his constitution has changed from a *Tae-eumin* to a *Soeumin.* Some also say that since women are generally shyer and less active than men, there are more women of *yin* constitutions and more men of *yang* constitutions. The statements above are incorrect. In addition, it is commonly thought that various living situations (the country, wilderness or a large city) and severe economic conditions (famine or war) will affect the constitution. This is also incorrect. The proportion of the Four Burners does not vary according to one's gender. Personality differences can be greatly influenced postnatally by social education and experiences.

6. Differentiating Methods of Sasang Constitutions

It was previously mentioned that SCM is a theory of self-rectification based on the constitution. Rectifying oneself through knowledge of others is the most effective method of self-cultivation and is the best way to provide service to others. By knowing the relationship between constitutional attributes and the desires of the mind, you can come to understand the mentality of others, as well as to cultivate your own nature. Moreover, to know others, it is necessary to understand their constitution since everyone has different constitutional attributes.

What are the constitutional characteristics of Sasang and how does one distinguish them? Dr. Lee Je-ma explained the method of differentiating the constitutions by using the Sasang (activity, mind, body and matter) method. The Sasang evolved out of the Two Modes (*yin-yang*). The Two Modes evolved out of *taichi.*

The Sasang method observes the activity, mind, body, and matter separately. "Activity" relates to all human activities. In *Longevity and Life Preservation in Eastern Medicine*, the foundation of heaven is called the "environmental frame" and when it manifests in social relationships it is called "human activities." Therefore, in the explanation of human activities, it states that *Taeyangins* are good at social acquaintances, *Soyangins* are good at appointed roles (the induction, organization and management of work), *Tae-eumins* are good at living quarters[11] and *Soeumins* are good at clanships. The concepts of appointed roles, social acquaintances, living quarters, and clanships are difficult to explain, for they are abstract eastern philosophical terms.

In simple terms, "human activities" indicates an innate talent

---

11) domestic environments.

of an individual constitution. This implies that talents vary across the constitutions. Therefore, the skills and talents mentioned in *Longevity and Life Preservation in Eastern Medicine* explain the abilities and inabilities of human activities.

The next method of differentiating the constitution is to observe "matter." Alcoholic drinks, sensual pleasure, money, and power are essentials in life. When people overindulge, they may ruin themselves and their families develop diseases. If there is a complete lack of these basic essentials, life will become miserable and bleak. Therefore, there has to be a balance.

If there is a moderate amount of drinking, sensual pleasure, money, and power, they will act as a fence, but if there is too much, they will become the walls of a jail. The point is that drinking, sensual pleasure, money and power exist as the essential matter or the materialistic environment. Observing the constitution from the aspect of "matter" is to grasp the relationship between the Sasang constitution and drinking, sensual pleasure, money, and power.

For instance, *Taeyangins* have a problem with drinking. This does not imply that *Taeyangins* drink excessively, but that they tend to use alcohol as a means to escape reality when they become indolent. Therefore, it is not correct to say that *Taeyangins* are heavy drinkers, but that they use alcohol to escape their indolent state. When they are out of balance, *Taeyangins* are too lazy to work and think only about drinking. In this state they visit bars frequently. This can lead to their ruin.

Taeyangins must be cautious of drinking, *Soyangins* must be cautious of sensual pleasure, *Tae-eumins* must be cautious of accumulating wealth, and *Soeumins* must be cautious of acquiring power. Alcohol, sensual pleasure, money and power are an essential part of life but each constitution has a weakness for one of them. It is obvious that those weaknesses can be avoided and each constitution must put forth the effort into doing so.

Expansion of knowledge, diligence, vigilance, and simplicity are the ways to control drinking, sensual pleasure, money, and power in one's daily life. These concepts will be explained later.

Such things belong to the concept of "matter." While the concept of "human activities" is about the merits or demerits of each constitution, the concept of "matter" is about the environmental factors that can affect one's life. Dr. Lee Je-ma's book then explains the subject of "mind and body" in considerable detail.

The most important detail of this subject is the theory of disease syndromes. Dr. Lee Je-ma explained mind and body by defining the states of mind and the physical condition in terms of health, mild disease, and serious disease. The most important thing to understand is that each constitution manifests particular constitutional disease syndromes. *Taeyangin*, *Soyangin*, *Tae-eumin* and *Soeumin* each have independent disease syndromes. Syndrome Medicine takes any symptom as an indication of a disease state. In SCM, however, a symptom can indicate a disease state for one constitution or a sign of health in another constitution. Again, different constitutions have different disease syndromes. Thus, in SCM, a disease syndrome becomes a constitutional disease syndrome.

Therefore, it is possible to diagnose a constitution through the disease syndromes. In other words, if the disease syndromes of a *Tae-eumin* are present, the person is a *Tae-eumin* and if the disease syndromes of a *Soeumin* are present, the person is a *Soeumin*.

Constitutional differentiation may appear simple, but it can become complicated if we lose sight of Dr. Lee Je-ma's basic theory. What has been presented thus far regarding physical shape, mental nature and disease syndromes describes the typical paradigm of each constitution. However, you are not likely to see a patient with a fixed mental state or one with a unique disease syndrome. Therefore, it is best to combine the three methods of analysis (physical shape, mental nature and disease syndromes) when possible. Each method has its own limitations and exceptions for constitutional differentiation.

Let's consider *mental nature*. Dr. Lee Je-ma's theory clearly states the unique characteristics of each constitution's consistant state of mind. In practice, however, it is hard to determine mental states because of the difference in the degree of cultivation and self-rectification a patient has achieved in suppressing desires. Knowing that the mind and personality change postnatally, this method could provide differing results over time. In addition, any attempt to measure mental characteristics is compromised by the current state of mind. A patient's present experience influences their response to questions. They appear more pessimistic or optimistic based on their current degree of sorrow, anger, joy, or pleasure.

The *disease syndrome method* is very accurate if a patient is experiencing a disease syndrome unique to a specific constitution. However, this does not happen frequently. Usually patients seek relief from chronic back pain, headaches or stomach pain; all of which can be experienced by all four constitutions.

Casual observation of a person's *physical shape* may lead to false conclusions. The combination of clothes and colors can give a false perception of the natural shape of the body. Both men and women often create their wardrobes in an attempt to hide unshapely physical characteristics.

In addition, the degree of development of the upper-body compared to the lower-body could be a deciding factor in determining a *Taeyangin* from a *Soyangin*. Without taking the time to accurately measure the difference between the upper and lower burner, constitutions may be misdiagnosed.

If this all sounds very confusing we need to reflect on Dr. Lee Je-ma's basic SCM theory and principle: "The constitutions are congenital and do not change over time. The sizes of the organs are predetermined from the time of birth. However, the personality develops postnatally and is variable."

This was discussed previously in Section 5 of Chapter 4.

If you thoroughly understand these three methods and limitations, you should be able to differentiate constitutions without making any mistakes. Otherwise, your differentiation will be made in haste. In addition, if you only superficially understand the explanations of constitutional characters in

Longevity and Life Preservation in Eastern Medicine and do not truly understand their profound meaning, you will run into trouble.

In my opinion, people who practice Eastern medicine misunderstand the Sasang constitutions. This is understandable because Dr. Lee Je-ma's writings are very abstruse and research has been lacking since his passing. Thus, I am advocating further clinical research for the advancement of SCM.

While the philosophical background of the *Inner Classic (Nei Jing)* is based on *yin-yang* and the Five-Element Theory, SCM is based on the Sasang philosophy, which has a strong relationship to Reformed Confucianism. Therefore, it needs to be accepted and studied as a new concept. It is not appropriate to interpret SCM using the theories of Syndrome Medicine. SCM should be studied and researched in its own way.

To understand SCM, one must understand its philosophical basis, which can be found in the book *Manuscript of Science.* Many who practice SCM avidly read *Longevity and Life Preservation in Eastern Medicine* to the point that they almost have the book memorized. Many people are not even aware that *Manuscript of Science* exists. This leads to an interpretation of SCM through the theories of Syndrome Medicine, rather than through the philosophy of *Manuscript of Science.* So, constitutions are determined only by relating disease symptoms to the various constitutions. For instance, someone with digestive problem is considered to be a *Soeumin*, while another person appears to be a *Tae-eumin* because he or she catches colds easily and has heart problems. Still another with low back pain and frequent urination is thought to be a *Soyangin.* Your first inclination may be incorrect unless you closely follow Dr. Lee Je-ma's theory and principle.

These constitutions are then given Sasang prescriptions instead of the traditional formulas used in TCM. This is a classic example of how those who practice TCM manage SCM. SCM needs its own systematic approach.

7. The Mental Nature of Sasang Constitution

Taeyangins always push forward without looking back. They want to move forward in all matters without observing their situations or their surroundings. This causes a state of urgency in *Taeyangins* and they always feel as though they are being chased or are under great pressure. Thus, the constant state of mind in *Taeyangins* is urgency.

Tae-eumins tend toward stillness. Since they do not like to move, they know the boundaries of their inner world but not the outside world. Also they have a good understanding of their domestic affairs but not the social world. As a result, they are uneasy with the outside world. This manifests as fear. *Tae-eumins* have more fear than the other constitutions and this fear is the constant state of mind in *Tae-eumins*.

Soyangins are always in a hurry to create new things. They always want to begin new projects and participate in new activities, but they have trouble finishing what they start. Thus, they know the outside world well but do not have a handle on their domestic affairs. Because their focus is on outside work, they do not have any interest in domestic work. Therefore, uneasiness toward their inner world arises. This manifests as anxiety, which is the constant state of mind of *Soyangins*.

Soeumins tend to remain in one place and do not have a tendency to go outside. This implies that *Soeumins* want stability. They do not necessarily tend to stay still like *Tae-eumins*, yet they do not want to go out. Then what is the difference between staying still and remaining in one place? From the viewpoint of "activity, mind, body, and matter," *Tae-eumins* are subject to "matter" while *Soeumins* are subject to the "body." This implies that *Soeumins* are hindered by the "body" while *Tae-eumins* are hindered by "matter" when attempting to move out of their inherent stillness.

Body and matter exist in a physical realm, while activity and mind exist metaphysically. Thus, *Taeyangins* and *Soyangins* are idealistic and impractical, in contrast to *Tae-eumins* and *Soeumins* who are realistic. *Tae-eumins* and *Soeumins* are realists who prioritize practical matters, i.e. how much they earn and spend for their families, whereas *Taeyangins* and *Soyangins* are idealists who live their lives according to their impractical dreams.

Taeyangins and *Soyangins* are less bound to matters such as money or property than the *yin* constitutions. For example, if they see a poor person, they will give them things such as clothes and money regardless of their own difficulties at that time. They simply follow their altruistic feelings. In the same situation, *Soeumins* and *Tae-eumins* react differently and will first calculate the profit and loss involved in a situation before they will help another person, regardless of the other person's poverty. *Soeumins* and *Tae-eumins* will not only consider their own situation, but also that of their kin, regional relations, as well as, how they will be treated after they help.

Generally, *Soeumins* are the opposite of *Taeyangins*. *Taeyangins* are very positive and active whereas *Soeumins* are passive. *Soeumins*' passive nature is such that they will not attempt something that no one has tried before. Thus, *Soeumins* have a nervous mind.

The urgent, fearful, anxious and nervous minds are considered the "constant states of mind" of the Sasang constitutions. The constant state of mind is not a disease condition; rather it is a particular mental nature of the individual's constitution. The disease is the next step.

There are also difficulties in determining a constitution through mental characteristics because one's true nature becomes diluted through education and self-refinement in a social environment. In this case, the patient may be surprised or angered to induce a reaction consistent with his or her true nature. Of course, this technique would be impractical in a doctor's office and would not conform to current ethical standards.

In the latter part of Chosun dynasty when Dr. Lee Je-ma lived, it was very difficult to diagnose a woman's constitution because doctors were limited to touch on a woman's body and could only palpate the pulse. Therefore, Dr. Lee Je-ma, while assessing the constitution of a woman, would surprise her by suddenly lifting her skirt. In Dr. Lee Je-ma's time, this type of a behavior would cause such embarrassment and disgrace that it would be considered a very serious crime. Regardless, Dr. Lee Je-ma would observe a woman's behavior at the moment her skirt was lifted to understand her true nature.

Another example would be commanding a large dog to suddenly bite a person. The person's reactions would be closely related to his or her nature. While *Tae-eumin* would be thrown into a state of chaos and faint, *Soeumin* would step by step calculate an escape strategy. *Soyangin* would fight with the dog without considering the danger while *Taeyangin* would first attempt to find a barrier to escape, and if this were not possible he would try to find an object to strike the dog and if none were available he would stop the dog from biting by forcing his fist into the dog's throat. Such behaviors are not acquired through education but follow the true nature of these people's mind. This example reflects the human survival instinct, not the constitutional differentiations.

In addition to surprising an individual, a constitution can be assessed by inviting a person to perform a certain task. For example, having a person move a large amount of firewood from one place to another will show the person's nature. A *Soyangin*, in his urgency, will simply throw the firewood from one place to another without moving himself. A *Taeyangin* would question whether it is necessary to move the wood and if it needs to be moved at this time. A *Tae-eumin* trusts his strength and will move a bunch of firewood at a time exerting a great deal of effort. A *Soeumin* will slowly move one or two pieces of firewood each time. Although this method works well for a *Soeumin* and he thinks that he is working efficiently, it will look weak and foolish to others. Thus, work style also depends on the nature of an individual temperament.

The nature of the mind is an important criterion that reflects the constitution but it can be distorted by various factors such as education, environment and mental cultivation. If the mental state is not controlled properly, it can adversely affect a person's total health and well-being.

Taeyangins anger easily. They lack patience and express their anger without consideration for how others may feel or how they will look. Therefore, they seem cold-blooded in the eyes of others. This is in fact due to their hastiness to accomplish their goals and their nature of being satisfied only after expressing their anger rather than settling it. This is the urgent nature of *Taeyangins*.

They can easily fall into delusions of grandeur and dream about an idealistic state rather than living in their present reality. For example, most people would be able to imagine how they would spend or share one million dollars if they had it. *Taeyangins*, however, like to immerse themselves in their very specific and detailed imaginations, from which they derive great pleasure.

One major fault of *Taeyangins* is that they will not see that they made mistakes when they fail. They will not think that their plan was impractical or unreasonable from the start. They invent all sorts of excuses but accept no blame. Instead, they will believe that their plan was not followed correctly and will place all the blame on others. They will believe that they are right until the bitter end. Therefore, unable to restrain their emotions, *Taeyangins* get upset if they do not have the proper support or understanding from others around them. If the situation worsens, they will lose their tempers more frequently.

In contrast to the quick-tempered and expressive *Taeyangins*, when *Soyangins* are agitated they suddenly fall into a state of depression. As a *yang* type, *Soyangins* are generally joyful, cooperative and sociable, but when their mental and emotional natures become unbalanced, they suddenly become depressed. They become sorrowful and melancholic and can feel as though they no longer want to live.

In general people of *yang* constitutions express their inner feelings outwards, but in an unbalanced state, *Soyangins* hold sadness in their hearts. This is a case of a *yang* person manifesting the nature and emotions of a *yin* person. This is not a positive change. *Taeyangins* become more unbalanced when they express their fury while *Soyangins* become more unbalanced when they hold sadness in their hearts.

So what about *Tae-eumins*? Generally *Soeumins* and *Tae-eumins* are *yin* persons in nature, so they speak modestly. Normally, they do not flaunt themselves. However, when *Tae-eumins* become anxious or restless in a pathological or psychological way, they desire to show off. Therefore, they fall into a state of "unrestrained pleasure" in which there is unlimited extravagance, recreation and sensual pleasures. For example, if a *Tae-eumin* were to become a millionaire overnight, he would buy expensive cars, expensive collections of books and clothes in order to show himself off to people and would not be able to keep or manage his newfound wealth. Such "unrestrained pleasure" is the characteristic of unbalanced *Tae-eumins*. Since *Tae-eumins* are *yin* persons, they should conform to characteristics that are *yin* in nature. If they have uncommon desires to flaunt themselves, it is an abnormal and unhealthy sign.

So how do *Soeumins*' characteristics appear? *Soeumins* are generally passive and introverted. They do not generally initiate conversation and give short answers when people talk to them. However, when their mental nature becomes unbalanced, they continue to talk even when they have not been asked any questions and will suddenly feel fluctuating joy (happy then sad) for no reason much like an insane person. When such urgency occurs in *Soeumins*, it is not a good sign.

Normal mental states appearing in abnormal ways indicate that there is an imbalance in the person's psychological state. This will result in disease if it is not corrected. Constitutional disease syndromes of the Sasang constitutions are therefore explained through a comparison of physical and mental states in a normal state, during a state of mild disease and in the case of serious disease.

8. Healthy Conditions and Constitutional Disease Syndromes of Each Constitution

Let's look at the healthy states of each constitution prior to discussing constitutional disease syndromes. As mentioned in the previous chapter, each body type has a state of health in which it is free from disease. *Tae-eumins* are healthy when they can perspire a great deal and *Soeumins* are healthy if their digestion is sound. *Soyangins* are healthy if they are not suffering from constipation and *Taeyangins* are healthy if they can urinate freely.

Under the circumstances mentioned above, the corresponding constitutions are physically healthy. The previous sections discussed the constant state of mind associated with each constitution. So we see that, mentally, there is a constant state of mind and physically, there is a state of health that is free from disease. Together they are the standards of health for each constitution.

So, what type of disease affects each constitution when the state of health breaks down? How does disease occur? And which treatment principle should be applied to treat it?

Mild disease occurs when the conditions that maintain health break down. For example, if *Tae-eumins* develop a mild disease, they will not sweat even when they should be. Normally, *Tae-eumins* break a sweat easily regardless of the temperature. They can even sweat during the winter while they are eating. If *Tae-eumins* feel tired or heavy, they should go to a sauna and sweat. If they try to sweat but cannot, they most likely have a disease.

A disease state for *Soeumins* is one in which they have diarrhea or sweat profusely. *Soyangins* have a disease if they suffer from constipation. And if *Taeyangins* are vomiting, or regurgitate saliva, or feel nauseous, they have a disease. These are the conditions in which a mild disease occurs from a breakdown of the healthy state.

When a mild disease worsens, a serious disease develops. For *Tae-eumins*, dysentery develops. This is not dysentery caused by bacterial infection, rather it is indicative of Irritable Bowel Syndrome. Here, psychological anxiety brings about alternating constipation and diarrhea with a feeling of fullness and uneasiness in the lower abdomen. This disease state is more complex if there is an absence of sweating in the initial stages followed by Irritable Bowel Syndrome. If the *Tae-eumins*' constant state of mind (fear) becomes extreme, then they will experience severe palpitations. When these severe palpitations occur and there is a fullness of the Large Intestine and an absence of sweating, the *Tae-eumin* constitution is in a severe state of disease.

The severe stage of disease for *Soeumins* is when they have diarrhea and their abdomen feels as cold as ice. *Soeumins* have naturally cold bodies. Once they develop digestive problems with accompanying coldness in their lower abdomens, they will have frequent episodes of diarrhea. This is a severe disease condition for *Soeumins*.

When *Soyangins* suffer from constipation for two days with no bowel movement, they feel a hot and stifling sensation in the chest. This is a bodily manifestation for an inability to withstand constipation. When constipation lasts for two to three days, the stifling sensation in the chest becomes a more severe problem than the constipation. Thus, constipation in *Soyangins* will result in stagnation and an uncomfortable sensation in the chest. When this develops, it is an inauspicious sign.

Dysphagia, called *yulgyuk*, is the sign of a serious disease for *Taeyangins*. It is a situation in which *Taeyangins* vomit frequently or are foaming from the mouth, or have dry heaves, or nausea, so that either no food can be swallowed or any food that is swallowed is vomited rather than digested.

Although it may be difficult to understand, let's take examples of *Taeyangins* and *Tae-eumins* in regards to the constitutional disease syndromes.

Taeyangins may fall prey to *Lumbar Vertebrae Disease induced by Exopathogen* and *Small Intestine Disease induced by*

Endopathogen. A disease induced by an exopathogen is one that develops on the surface of the body or the skin. It is considered an exterior disease. A disease induced by an endopathogen is related to the internal organs and is an interior disease.

So, what is *Lumbar Vertebrae Disease induced by Exopathogen* specifically?

Taeyangins have weak lower bodies but strong rising energy. That is why they have a weakness in their lower limbs. This situation will bring about *haeyuk.* In *haeyuk*, there are few problems in the upper body but the lower body is too weak to walk well. This is called *Lumbar Vertebrae disease.*

To treat the *Lumbar Vertebrae Disease induced by Exopathogen*, the rising energy must be pulled down. To do this, the most important thing is to control the temper, especially the anger. An herbal prescription is the next step. If *Taeyangins* continue to get angry, they will further accelerate the rising energy. In this case, no medicine will be useful. Before taking a prescription, *Taeyangins* have to attempt to refrain from sadness and anger and keep their minds calm. In addition, they should avoid greasy foods. If *Taeyangins* eat a lot of foods that are high in nutrition in order to boost their energy, their excessive rising energy will develop into heat. Therefore, overly nutritious, hot, spicy and greasy foods should be avoided and instead foods that are energetically clear and have a bland taste such as fruits, vegetables, and seafoods should be ingested to descend energy. Foods that are easy to digest, pass through the body quickly, and facilitate urination are appropriate for *Taeyangins.*

Small Intestine Disease induced by Endopathogen is known as *yulgyuk* or dysphagia. In SCM, the Lungs and Liver are the gateways through which *qi* and Fluids are gathered or dispersed, and each organ alternates in carrying out this function. So in this disease, the Small Intestine, which belongs to the Liver system (Lower-Middle Burner), has insufficient energy to absorb *yin-cold qi*, while the warm *qi* in the Esophagus, which belongs to the Lung system (Upper Burner), becomes exuberant. When this occurs, the dispersing *qi* of the Esophagus is excessive while the gathering *qi* of Lower-Middle Burner is weak. Thus, the food cannot enter the body and is vomited instead. This is what is called *yulgyuk* or dysphagia.

Diseases in *Taeyangins* result from their strong rising *qi* and weak gathering and accumulating *qi*. In general, *Taeyangins* are healthy but they can suddenly fall ill from *haeyuk* or *yulgyuk* or both simultaneously in a single day. This is the distinguishing factor between *Taeyangins* and *Soeumins*. *Soeumins* will show signs of fatigue and a dislike of speaking or moving due to a lack of *qi*, at the initial stage of a disease. In contrast, *Taeyangins* develop disease suddenly in a single day without any signs. Therefore, diseases can be said to develop according to people's constitutions.

Taeyangins must first pay attention to weight gain because they should have proper elimination to maintain clear *yang qi*. If they become overweight, internal heat is created due to a stagnation of *qi*. Secondly, their complexion should be light. The reason is the same as above. Thirdly, there should be no problem with urination. Fourthly, the epigastric region should not have any hard masses. If there is a mass in that region, the greater the size the more serious the disease.

For the treatment of *Taeyangins*, other things are more important than herbal prescriptions. Dr. Lee Je-ma's book states, "Be cautious of deep sorrow and sudden anger," and "Be wary of anger and eat plain foods." This implies that the control of emotions should be primary and foods that are greasy and pungent should not be ingested in order to augment Liver *yin*, after which herbal prescriptions should be applied. As for the foods, frequent ingestion of delicacies, high cholesterol foods, and pungent and hot foods cause a chronic accumulation of heat that in turn brings about diseases in *Taeyangins*. So for *Taeyangins*, you should not think in terms of preventing their illnesses with herbal tonics but rather focus on controlling their emotions and foods and if disease still develops, then use herbal prescriptions.

The disease syndromes of *Tae-eumins* consist of *Exterior Cold Disease induced from the Esophagus affected by Cold* and *Interior Febrile Disease induced from the Liver affected by*

Heat.

Tae-eumins have a large Liver and small Lungs. A large Liver indicates strong gathering *qi* while small Lungs indicate weak dispersing *qi*. Since there is an excess of gathering *qi* with deficiency of dispersing *qi*, *Tae-eumin* diseases are eventually caused by the large Liver and small Lungs.

Then how do *Exterior Cold Disease* and *Interior Febrile Disease* develop?

In contrast to the *Taeyangins*, *Tae-eumins* have small Lungs and a large Liver. Therefore, *Tae-eumins* can easily accumulate heat inside as their physiology continually accumulates *qi* without dispersing it. Here, the lack of dispersing *qi* is the *Exterior Cold Disease* while the excess of gathering *qi* is the *Interior Febrile Disease. Interior Febrile Disease* is followed by constipation and *Exterior Cold Disease* has an absence of sweating. This is similar to diseases in which there is fever without sweating such as typhoid fever and the flu.

The treatment principle of the *Exterior Cold Disease* is to promote sweating, while that of the *Interior Febrile Disease* is to cool the interior heat through urination and bowel movements.

Ultimately, since either the small Lungs or the large Liver of *Tae-eumins* cause their diseases, if the two syndromes that arise from these organs are treated, all *Tae-eumin* diseases will be included in the treatment. This principle is also applicable to the other constitutions.

If we compare *Tae-eumins* and *Soyangins*, their disease syndromes will develop from *Exterior Cold Disease* into *Interior Febrile Disease. Soyangins*' diseases develop due to *fire* and *heat* while *Tae-eumins*' diseases develop from *dryness*. That is why the word "dryness" is always included in the explanation of *Tae-eumins*' diseases. The dryness that comes from the lack of dispersing *qi* is released by inducing sweat and the dryness that comes from the strong gathering *qi* can be released by promoting bowel movements.

Eventually, irrespective of *Exterior Cold* or *Interior Febrile Diseases* in *Tae-eumins*, the treatment principle is to promote sweating and bowel movements. For *Tae-eumins*, it is useless to tonify blood. The reason why deer horn is used for *Tae-eumins* is to control the dryness, which can be considered as a deficient symptom that occurs due to the conflict between the Righteous *qi* and the pathogenic *qi*.

Soeumins have large Kidneys and a small Spleen. Their syndromes are also divided into two: *Exterior Febrile Disease induced from the Kidney affected by Heat* and *Interior Cold Disease induced from the Stomach affected by Cold*. In contrast, *Soyangins* have a large Spleen and small Kidneys. Their syndromes are classified into the *Exterior Cold Disease induced from the Spleen affected by Cold* and *the Interior Febrile Disease induced from the Stomach affected by Heat.*

As previously mentioned, certain diseases easily afflict certain constitutions. Although everyone can catch a cold, develop abdominal pain or liver disease, it is vital to know the weaknesses of the constitutions and which types of diseases warrant caution. Furthermore, it would be beneficial to be able to associate the state of health, mild disease and serious disease with the particular weakness of a constitution. If these things are considered carefully, it will become easy to understand how individual weaknesses predispose one to certain diseases. This cannot be accomplished by thoughtless rote memorization of predispositions because that will not lead to the proper understanding of the constitutional disease syndromes nor their practical application.

For example, *Tae-eumins* are usually overweight and have a voracious appetite. Moreover they are too lazy to exercise so they gain weight easily. Eventually, they can become obese, develop hypertension and problems in the circulatory system or have a stroke. To treat this type of person it is less important to prescribe medication than it is to ensure that they can urinate, have bowel movements, and sweat regularly by instigating changes in their diet and lifestyle as well as encouraging daily exercises. In addition, it is important to attempt to modify their narrow worldview into one that is more progressive and enterprising. This behavior modification will be just as important in treating their disease processes. And although beef and deer horn are said to be good for *Tae-eumins*, if they ingest these foods and do not exercise they will find themselves in serious trouble.

The principles of SCM tend to be frequently misunderstood. As previously mentioned, people often think that recommending deer horn and beef to *Tae-eumins* is simple and convenient way to use SCM. But it is a mistake to think that deer horn and beef will make *Tae-eumins* healthy.

So why are people so easily persuaded into following this type of misdirection? People like convenience and do not like to change their lifestyles and diets. They would prefer to take one or two herbs or foods to supplement their diets. The intention of SCM, however, is quite different from this view. The SCM recommendations given to each constitution consist of very narrow choices. Simply memorizing those things that are beneficial for each constitution without gaining a thorough understanding of the entire concept of SCM will prove to be insufficient.

There are several important factors in the treatment of disease. SCM is a self-generating constitutional medicine that stems from a mode of thought that is derived from Confucianism rather than one that supports Syndrome Medicine. The treatment principle of SCM is based upon the view that SCM is primarily a "differentially-responding medicine." Until the introduction of constitutional medicine, eastern doctors believed that all human bodies were the same. However, *yin* and *yang* constitutions respond differently to herbal medicines. Therefore, the method of observing disease syndromes should naturally also come from this differential point of view.

Secondly, SCM is a "self-regulating medicine." This is a crucial concept because of the fact that the proper prescription is not the only thing that is needed to cure a disease. It is also important to observe a person's response and make adjustments to the prescription. This will be indispensable to the healing process. Some people will have a very good response to a prescription while others will not have much of a response. For example, *yang* persons will have a very quick response but *yin* persons will need long-term use of a prescription. In this way, disease follows the character of each constitution. A *yang* person will develop diseases that occur suddenly and worsen quickly, while a *yin* person will develop diseases that occur gradually and worsen slowly. Therefore, in treating a disease, the self-regulation processes of the individual constitutions must be taken into careful consideration and prescriptions must be made according to the response they will elicit in each constitution.

Western medicine is a "cause-eliminating medicine." For example, if a patient presents with pneumonia, the western medical establishment will prescribe antibiotics to attempt to kill bacteria, such as streptococcus. In contrast, Eastern medicine is an "environment-regulating medicine." Eastern medicine will not attempt to aggressively exterminate bacteria; rather they will be left alone. They are allowed to stay in the body and will gradually disappear by themselves through regulating the environment that they live in. In short, by applying syndrome differentiation, bacteria can be eliminated. However, SCM not only applies syndrome differentiation, it also applies "constitutional" syndrome differentiation. Therefore, SCM is a self-regulating medicine and a "Constitutional" Syndrome Medicine.

To this day there is a uniformed and schematic view of disease that encourages systematic treatment of disease. One disease is treated in one certain way. However, people are individually unique, and so under a schematic view of medicine, certain disease will be curable and certain others will not be curable. Those that are incurable are given the label "psychosomatic." This term, however, is frequently misused. Many of these "incurable" cases could be effectively treated using self-regulating medical techniques, but since they are treated with cause-eliminating medical techniques, they do not respond. This is found to be true particularly with chronic diseases, geriatric diseases, psychosomatic diseases, and psychiatric diseases.

There exist treatment methods that are appropriate for each and every disease. Thus there are many cases in which western medicine, Eastern medicine or SCM would be the most advantageous method to use depending upon the response of the disease. It would be beneficial to think about why we need Eastern medicine and SCM, and why Eastern medicine and western medicine should complement one another.

Since the disease syndromes of the Sasang constitutions in Dr. Lee Je-ma's book are so abstruse and peculiar, even people with knowledge of Syndrome Medicine have trouble understanding them. The purpose of this book is not to present the technical knowledge of SCM. Instead, it is to give a general introduction and present the basic principles of Sasang Constitutional Medicine.

<Note>

It seems appropriate to introduce the disease syndromes of each constitution up to this level for the general reader. However, for those readers who are particularly interested in the theory of differential syndromes, see <Appendix 1: Theories of Constitutional Disease Syndromes> at the end of this book. This will provide additional information to those who have technical knowledge of Eastern medicine.

9. Daily Wisdom to Achieve Health and Longevity

Sasang constitutions have individually specific characteristics and health conditions. This must be taken into consideration and attention must be paid to lifestyle and diet in order to acquire the key to longevity. Additionally, a thorough understanding of the strengths and weaknesses of an individual's character and an earnest endeavor to supplement and improve these weaknesses can lead one down the path of self-realization.

I will again reiterate the characteristics of the four constitutions. *Taeyangins* are highly intelligent and extremely creative, encompassing many personalities that are heroic and brave. They are self-righteous, masculine, highly active and progressive. However, they lack planning, act without restraint, and do not know the meaning of the word "retreat." They communicate well with others, regardless of whether or not they know them, but are easily angered when things do not turn out to their liking.

Tae-eumins are honest, taciturn and act in trustworthy manner. They are persistent and have great patience. They are generally conservative in nature and dislike change. Though *Tae-eumins* may look dignified, they are also highly suspicious, and are arrogant and greedy. They place priority on their domestic affairs but not on outside affairs. They dislike exercising and speaking, but enjoy recreational activities. They also carry a great deal of fear and have a tendency to be lazy.

Soyangins are very active, passionate, and hot-tempered. They like to sacrifice themselves in order to help others, and are righteous and straightforward. They act hastily but are kind and are unconcerned about profit and loss when helping others. They pay more attention to outside work and tend to neglect their own or family work. They begin work easily but have trouble finishing things they have started. They lack persistence and get bored easily, and so they may begin many projects without completing them.

Soeumins are docile, calm and sociable. They are witty and meticulous, and plan and organize things well. They are generally introverted and shy and do not easily express their thoughts or feelings to others. They are passive and thus lack the drive to begin things. They are subject to gains and losses, and do not like being interfered with in their affairs. They hold a lot of jealousy and do not easily forget when others hurt their feelings.

In terms of the mental desires for each constitution, *Taeyangins* have self-indulgence, *Tae-eumins* have greed, *Soyangins* have partiality, and *Soeumins* have idleness. These desires belong to the category of "activity," while those that belong to "matter" are described in the chapter, "*A Discourse on General Health Maintenance*," in Dr. Lee Je-ma's book. That chapter relays information about the wisdom of life to promote long and healthy living.

Each constitution has a different guiding principle to follow in order to perfect one's character. Conducting oneself in a saintly manner is not enough because there are vast psychological differences among the constitutions. Thus temperamental warnings also differ. For example, *Soyangins* have a talent for "appointed roles" but not for "living quarters." Therefore, *Soyangins* should not live their lives based on their sensual desires. It is because of their sensual lives that they have problems with "living quarters." So *Soyangins* must live a life of simplicity. In contrast, *Tae-eumins* should not develop a liking for extravagance and material wealth. They must learn to listen and observe the outer world.

Each constitution should pay careful attention to the attitudes and behaviors of simplicity, the expansion of knowledge, diligence and vigilance. Simplicity implies living a simple, moderate, non-complicated life. There are four important keys to living either a longer or shorter life. Extravagance, greed, laziness, and urgency will cause a shortened life span. Simplicity, the expansion of knowledge, diligence and vigilance will lead to longevity. The former and the latter have a polar relationship. Therefore, to avoid the former, the latter should be practiced.

In the case of *Soyangins*, how can they avoid sensual pleasures? Living a sensual life implies that they are excessively arrogant and lead an extravagant life. Thus, sensual life refers to not only one's sexual life but also, in a greater sense, to an extravagant and prodigal life. For this constitution, simplicity and moderation are the best medicine.

Tae-eumins are fond of material wealth. This implies that they are only capable of finding comfort in their present reality since they engross themselves in money making and gathering material wealth. When *Tae-eumins* find comfort in their present reality, they believe that what they see in their narrow world is everything, similar to the frog-in-a-well mentality. So for them, the material goods that they see in front of them are the only valuable things in the world. In order to avoid such a narrow-minded mentality, they have to listen to the information from the outer world. Listening and observing indicate gaining knowledge and experience from the outside world through reading books, listening to the news or taking trips.

Taeyangins have to refrain from drinking. Why? Generally, in an unbalanced state, *Taeyangins* are lazy. They do not work diligently and when they are working, they easily fall into narcissism. If their work is progressing well, they drink because they feel good. If they have trouble in their work, they still drink because they feel bad. Instead of earnestly making an effort to find the cause of the problem, they get angry and look for a way out in alcohol. If they are drunk, they feel as though everything in the world seem to be going their way. Because they indulge in alcohol, their narcissistic behavior worsens and they become less conscious of everyone around them and work only when they feel up to it. In this way, they become even lazier. Therefore, they must strive to be more diligent.

Soeumins have an affinity for authoritative power. Those who like authoritative power obviously like to make factions and cannot embrace everyone equally. Regardless of the amount of power they have, *Soeumins* want to keep their power and tend to use or perhaps abuse others. Power and authority are easily abused. Therefore, *Soeumins* have to be careful when they have power because it will not last forever and it may be used against them in the future. That is why they must be cautious. *Soeumins* tend to get very competitive over trivial things so that they do not easily yield to others. A *Soeumin* with this attitude can easily misuse his or her power and become a dictator, and this can lead to self-destruction. Therefore, in order to avoid such a mishap, *Soeumins* must respect people who are wiser and always be cautious with their conduct.

In truth, the situations described above were applied to the four constitutions in "*A Discourse on the General Health Maintenance*." However, they were applied specifically to the four types of people: the person who lives in the mountain, the person who lives in the city, the intellectual, and the peasant.

The person who lives in the mountain has to listen and observe in order to expand his knowledge of the outer world (the world outside his district) and achieve longevity. The person who lives in the city has to have simplicity and moderation in order to achieve longevity. The intellectual has to practice vigilance in order to achieve longevity. And the peasant in the countryside has to be diligent in order to achieve longevity.

One must avoid luxury and sensual pleasure to be simple and moderate. To be diligent, one must avoid drinking and sensual pleasure. One must avoid authoritative power to be vigilant. And one must be free from material wealth to be able to listen and observe the outer world in order to gain knowledge. This is the wisdom of a healthy life. Though this may seem like a discussion on ethics without any relation to medicine, isn't it important to maintain these attitudes in order to lead a healthy life?

It is the view of SCM that human beings are not perfect. If human beings were born perfect, perhaps there would be no meaning to life. Life may be the process of painstakingly resolving problems that arise from being imperfect since birth. The person who is balanced in *yin-yang* does not need to cultivate himself and because of that may lose the meaning of life. Human beings are destined to live and adapt their lives with society and nature. Thus this is the problem of how we can adapt our true nature to practical reality.

The fact that human beings were born imperfect indicates that there is a physical imperfection in the size of their organs and a psychological imbalance in their constant state of mind and desire. Therefore, if we first understand ourselves physically and psychologically, and by complementing our weaknesses and cultivating ourselves to accumulate true knowledge and proper conduct, we can all elevate ourselves to the level of a sage.

In other words, it is not good to live without correcting our weaknesses. It would be very unfortunate for a *Soyangin* or a *Soeumin* to keep his or her mental nature until death. In the view of SCM, the ideal life is one in which people are able to adapt their character to everyday life by implementing methods of self-cultivation.

Frequently people say that two people who have the same personality traits will not have a good marriage. If that is true, then is a *Soyangin* husband better off with *Soeumin* wife? Obviously, getting married to a person of a different constitution can be advantageous since both people can complement each other. A *Soeumin* can learn the strengths of a *Soyangin* to improve herself while a *Soyangin* can learn to be like a *Soeumin* to perfect himself. In this way, they will help complete one another to become better human beings. However, if a *Soyangin* and a *Soeumin* always manifest their own characteristics without understanding one another, they will have many arguments and will eventually fall ill.

The reason we have jobs is to refine ourselves while working among different types of people and learn to live by adapting to the reality of society. Viewed this way, our job becomes a way to cultivate our character. It is very important to know the strengths and weaknesses of our bodies and minds when selecting a job. This means that by knowing and purifying one's true nature beforehand, one can select the proper means of livelihood.

Since *Soyangins* are fairly open-minded, they may be well suited to be diplomats. *Soeumins* are intellectual; therefore, they are well suited to being scientists or scholars. *Tae-eumins* are very shrewd and so they are well suited to being businessmen or politicians. *Taeyangins* are creative and communicate well with others. In addition they have strong leadership abilities. These skills would be an asset in such careers as computer analyst, general management, efficiency analyst, scientist or inventor. These statements make a certain amount of sense. In these situations, the strengths of the individual constitutions are being properly applied to their own advantage. They will surely benefit if their strengths are used in the right way, but if their strengths are misused, they will be faced with great troubles.

Tae-eumins always seem dignified and gentlemanly in the eyes of others. However, if they veer off in the wrong direction, they can become wicked intellectual criminals or swindlers.

Though they may look good on a superficial level, inside they can become treacherous persons who defraud others. All of the constitutions have merits that, when misused, convert into vices.

We can take another example from sporting activities. If there is a question of which event to choose when practicing sports, it will be proper to think in reverse. *Tae-eumins* and *Soeumins* have strong endurance. Marathon running or something that is performed for a long time is proper for *yin* constitutions. However, if an event requires quick movements or a quick sense of timing, *yang* constitutions will be better suited. Even though both *yang* and *yin* constitutions have their particular advantages, it is inadvisable to continuously practice those sports that allow their advantages to manifest. Their particular advantages in a given sport may help them set temporary records, but to look at the chosen sport as a method of maintaining health, it may not be suitable for balancing their bodies.

This principle also holds true for recreational activities. If you have a *yin* constitution, you should select an activity that is opposite to your constitution such as jogging, swimming or hiking (all outdoor activity) to broaden your horizons. Or if your lower body is more developed than your upper body, it will be better for you to perform exercises that strengthen your upper body. This is the method of self-cultivation through constitutional theory.

Generally, it would be better for *Soyangins* and *Taeyangins* to perform exercises to develop their lower bodies. *Tae-eumins* should choose exercises that will make them sweat, and *Soeumins* should choose exercises that are light and do not overly tax their bodies, such as yoga. This would be better for them than exercises that use up a lot of the body's energy over an extended amount of time, like weight training.

Chapter 5
Teachings on Health Cultivation by Dr. Lee Je-ma

Dr. Lee Je-ma explained his methods for healthy living in several chapters of *Manuscript of Science*, *The New Edition on the Salvation of People* and *Longevity and Life Preservation in Eastern Medicine*. This chapter quotes directly from several sections of these books in order to share Dr. Lee Je-ma's wisdom of how to live a healthy life with the reader.

Longevity and Life Preservation in Eastern Medicine consists of many chapters such as, "A Discourse on Nature and Order" "A Discourse on the Four Principles" "A Discourse on the Establishment and Supplement" "A Discourse on Viscera and Bowels" "A Discourse on the Origin of Eastern Medicine" and "A Discourse on Syndrome Differentiation." The chapter "A Discourse on General Health Maintenance" was originally written as a separate work but was later included as a part of this book. *Manuscript of Science* is a book of philosophy consisting of several themes including the "Summary of Confucianism," "Self- cultivation" and "Cautions on Insincerity." *The New Edition on the Salvation of People* consists of "A Discourse on Five Blessings," "Advice on Longevity," and "A Discourse on Proper Knowledge and Conduct."

This chapter contains several excerpts from *Longevity and Life Preservation in Eastern Medicine* and from *The New Edition on the Salvation of People*. For the sake of convenience, they have been summarized and not necessarily presented in their original texts. In addition, I have taken the liberty of extracting some sentences from their original paragraphs and added them to others.

"A Discourse on Viscera and Bowels" and "A Discourse on the Origin of Eastern Medicine" as well as the Theory of Syndrome Differentiation of the four constitutions and their prescriptions have been omitted due to their technical nature. Instead, certain sections of "A Discourse on General Health Maintenance," "A Discourse on Nature and Order," and "A Discourse on Establishment and Supplement" are discussed. "Advice on Longevity" from *The New Edition on the Salvation of People* is not introduced because of its similarity to "A Discourse on General Health Maintenance" and only certain parts of "A Discourse on Five Blessings" and "A Discourse on Proper Knowledge and Conduct" are mentioned.

Because there are many abstract passages in the original text, a direct translation would be difficult to understand. Therefore, the passages were simplified and their meanings clarified to make them more understandable to the reader. Utmost care has been given to insure that the original meanings and concepts of Dr. Lee Je-ma were not changed in this publication.

1. A Discourse on General Health Maintenance

This section will cover the contents of "A Discourse on General Health Maintenance." In these modern times there are many people whose only concerns are success and money. Because of this, these people may lose the true joy and value of life. They may also damage their health. Such people will be given the opportunity to reflect upon their values as they read each line.

1) Childhood Is Like a New Bud that Sprouts in the Spring

Childhood is a time when there is a yearning for knowledge

and information and a love and respect for others, similar to the sprouting of a bud in the spring. During young adulthood, one esteems bravery, has an open-heart and is quick to take action, much like young trees in the summer. Adulthood brings the enjoyment of making friends, gathering the fruits of one's efforts and the knowledge of self-cultivation and self-restraint like the harvesting of grains in autumn. Old age is a time when there is a strong desire towards systematic planning and secrets are kept like roots hidden under frozen ground in the winter.

A child who enjoys learning is greatly respected. A young adult who respects his or her elders is admired. An adult who knows how to love with an open mind is esteemed. And a person who knows how to protect what is righteous during his or her old age is a hero. A person with genuine talent and a kind heart is a true hero. However, there are people with genuine talents who do not have a kind heart!

Children's illnesses arise from a stagnation of the four emotions (sorrow, anger, joy and pleasure) stemming from a lack of information and knowledge, so they need to be cared for by their affectionate mother. Young adults get sick from a stagnation of the four emotions stemming from a lack of courage, so they need to be protected by their wise fathers or intelligent older brothers. During adulthood, help should come from a judicious younger brother or good friend. During old age, help should come from a filial son or grandson[12].

2) The Home of a Virtuous Person Attracts Other Virtuous People

The home of a virtuous person attracts other virtuous people whereas the home of an immoral person attracts other immoral people. A gathering of many virtuous people activates the virtuous energy of their organs while a gathering of many immoral people arouses the immoral energy of their minds.

12) a male descendant.

Immoral people gather in the houses where people are overindulging in drinking and sex, and are hungry for wealth and power. Thus their family offspring will become afflicted with diseases.

Factions and cliques will always gather in the house of people who thirst for authoritative power and intrigue. This will eventually destroy the family. The descendants of a family that likes money are arrogant and foolish, so they will lead to the collapse of the family.

In a house where no work is successful, family members are constantly getting sick, good and evil struggle with one another and troubles abound, the family will be on the verge of ruins. Only wise and affectionate parents and dutiful children will have the ability to manage the situation.

3) The Way to Longevity

Overindulgence, indolence, prejudice, and greed can shorten one's life span. The overindulgent person will surely engage in sensual pleasure. The lazy person will surely become addicted to drinking. The prejudiced person will surely fight for power. The greedy person will surely die in the pursuit of money.

In contrast, a person who is simple and exercises moderation will achieve longevity. So will a person who is diligent, a person who is vigilant and a person who knows how to listen and observe the outer world.

The person who is simple and moderate will avoid sensual pleasures; the diligent person will avoid drinking; the person who is vigilant will avoid the pursuit of authoritative power; and the person who knows how to listen and observe the outer world will avoid the pursuit of wealth.

Overindulgence in extravagance and sensual pleasures results in desolate living quarters. Drinking in excess leads to poor conduct and improper behavior. The fight for power causes a troubled mind. And a disorderly appointed role is due to the pursuit of wealth.

When a man respects a woman, sensual pleasures can be enjoyed in a responsible fashion. When a man loves his friends, even when they are drinking together he will have clear virtue. When a man respects a sage, he can utilize power appropriately. When a man cares for the poor, he will do great service with his wealth.

Overdrinking, sensual pleasure, wealth and power have been cautioned since ancient times as they were compared to the four walls of a jail. These four vices influence not only one's longevity and family fortune, but also the order of a society. Therefore, as long as a society does not succumb to these vices, it will closely resemble the era of King Yao and King Shun. (Yao and Shun were legendary emperors of the golden age, circa 24th-23rd century BC. They were sages of the highest virtue, integrity, and righteousness and were exalted by Confucius.)

In general, people must be simple and moderate, diligent, cautious and know how to listen and observe. A person with these four qualities will naturally achieve longevity. A person with three of these qualities will have a slightly shorter life span than one who has all four. A person with only two of these qualities will live a long life if he or she exercises respect but will die young if he or she is negligent.

4) Respect Will Lead to Longevity but Neglect Will Lead to a Short Life

In general, a respectful and diligent person will live long, while a negligent and greedy person will die young. A hungry person who eats food hastily will scatter the energy of his intestines. Sudden wealth will disturb the life of a poor person. Even though a person may be hungry, as long as he is content, the energy of his intestines will be in order. Even though a person may be poor, if he is peaceful, his life will be preserved.

Therefore, it is respectable to eat food to the level where

hunger is tolerable, rather than to greedily overeat. It is respectable to wear enough clothing so that the cold is tolerable, rather than to indulge in too many warm clothes. It is respectable to use one's physical strength for the proper amount of labor instead of living in idleness. It is respectable to gain one's property through diligent effort, instead of greedily waiting for an unexpected windfall.

5) A Person Who Lives in the Mountains Will Die Young If He Does Not Listen and Observe (to Gain Knowledge and Information)

A person who lives in the mountains will die young if he does not listen and observe (to gather knowledge and information). A person who lives in the city will die young if he does not live simply. A peasant in the countryside will die young if he lives without diligence. The intellectual will die young if he does not exercise vigilance.

If a person living in the mountains listens and observes (to gather knowledge and information) not only will he have a long and prosperous life, he will also be the most distinguished man in that region. If a person living in the city practices simplicity and moderation, not only will he have a long and prosperous life, he will also be the most admired man in the city. If a peasant living in the countryside is diligent, not only will he have a long and prosperous life, he will also be the most popular man in that area. And, if the intellectual exercises vigilance, not only will he have a long and prosperous life, he will also be the most revered man among the intellectuals.

6) The Mind of an Overindulgent Person Laughs at an Ordinary Life

A person who is extravagant cannot enjoy an ordinary life. He is arrogant, surrounds himself in luxuries, and makes light of domestic affairs. Because of this he does not understand the difficulties of earning a living. He is extremely unskilled and deceptive, so he will continually overindulge in sexual pleasures and luxuries, and he will not experience regret in his lifetime.

A lazy person has a mind that is rough and wild, so he does not want to work in a practical manner, and instead wastes his time on empty dreams. Since he is reluctant to be diligent, he drinks to avoid responsibility. This is a temporary measure he uses to avoid diligence. Since a person who uses alcohol to escape does not like physical labor, he has worries that are as great as mountains. A person who is blinded by lust suffers from anxieties that cut him like a knife. Such overindulgence in drinking and sexual pleasure breaks the spirit, while alcohol poisoning and sexual exhaustion attack the body. Together, they eventually bring about death.

2. A Discourse on Nature and Order

In this section, parts of "A Discourse on Nature and Order" from *Longevity and Life Preservation in Eastern Medicine* will be introduced.

Since ancient times, nature and humanity were considered to be one and the same. Nature was seen as the macrocosm while human beings were regarded as the microcosm. Human beings are born from the Great Earth, also known as Mother Nature. They form societies with their bodies and minds, which they inherited from nature and live in constant communication with nature.

"A Discourse on Nature and Order" represents Dr. Lee Je-ma's views on the cosmos and humanity.

1) Human Life Relies on Geographical, Hereditary, Social, and Temporal Factors

The four environmental frames are locality, human relationships, social relationships, and the times of heaven. The four types of human activities are living quarters, clanship, social acquaintances, and appointed roles. The times of heaven are eternal, society is enormous, family relations are extensive and geography is vast. Appointed roles should be in order, social acquaintances should be well established, clanship should be well arranged, and living quarters should be well regulated.

2) The Ears Hear the Times of Heaven and the Eyes Look upon Society

The ears hear the times of heaven, the eyes look upon society, the nose smells kinship, and the mouth tastes locality. It is easy to understand how the ears hear the times of heaven and the eyes look upon society. But how is it possible that the nose smells kinship and the mouth tastes locality? Couldn't smelling be described as sensing and recognizing people's expressions and moods, as well as, determining the wisdom of their individual abilities and behaviors? Can't tasting be described as experiencing many aspects of people's lifestyles while living in a certain locality?

3) The Head Represents Knowledge and Experience and the Shoulders Represent Dignity

The ears, eyes, nose, and mouth perceive the environment (They are the sense organs that receive and observe external phenomena). The Lungs, Spleen, Liver, and Kidneys establish human activities (They are the fundamental organs that allow human beings to perform their duties). The jaw, chest, navel and abdomen execute wisdom. The head, shoulders, waist, and hips carry out conduct.

First of all, in terms of the four internal organs, the Lungs correspond to appointed roles, the Spleen corresponds to social acquaintances, the Liver corresponds to clanship and the Kidneys correspond to living quarters.

Next, in terms of the jaw, chest, navel, and abdomen, human beings should have the four basic qualities of wisdom, administration, moderation, and generosity. The jaw represents wisdom, the chest symbolizes administration, the navel represents moderation and the abdomen symbolizes generosity. A wise person should not be arrogant. An administrative person should not be pretentious. A moderate person should not be cruel to others. And a generous person should not boast.

In terms of the head, shoulders, waist, and hips, the head represents discernment, the shoulders relate to nobility, the waist symbolizes talent, and the hips coincide with scheme. A discerning person should not deprive others of their share. A noble person should not indulge in extravagance. A talented person should not be lazy. And a scheming person should not pilfer. The discerning head contains self-indulgence. The noble shoulders embody extravagance. The talented waist has indolence. And the scheming hips hold greed. Self-indulgence refers to selfishness, extravagance refers to vanity, indolence refers to low self-esteem, and greed refers to pilfering.

4) The Ears, Eyes, Mouth, and Nose of Human Beings Delight in Virtue above All Else

(Although people have an affinity for virtue and an aversion to vice, simultaneously they have selfish and misguided motives.)

The ears delight in pleasant sounds, the eyes welcome beautiful colors, the nose enjoys sweet smells, and the mouth relishes good tastes. Pleasant sounds comfort the ears, beautiful colors enrich the eyes, sweet smells benefit the nose, and good tastes support the mouth.

The Lungs dislike noise, the Spleen dislikes ugly colors, the Liver dislikes foul odors, and the Kidneys dislike foul tastes. Noises are harsh on the Lungs, ugly colors are repelling to the Spleen, foul odors are unpleasant to the Liver and bad tastes are displeasing to the Kidneys.

(Human beings esteem virtue and detest vice, but selfishness and misguided actions exist in everyday knowledge and conduct. Because of this, human beings have contradicting intentions that they should be conscious of at all times.)

The ears, eyes, mouth, and nose of human beings have the greatest affinity for virtue while the Lungs, Spleen, Liver and Kidneys have the greatest aversion to vice. However, there is nothing more selfish than the jaw, chest, navel and abdomen, which represent knowledge, and nothing lazier than the head, shoulders, waist and hips, which represent conduct.

5) King Yao and King Shun Governed with Benevolence Five Thousand Years Ago

Even though it has been 5,000 years since King Yao and King Shun benevolently governed the people, they are still held up to be symbols of virtue and integrity, demonstrating the magnitude of people's affinity for virtue. Even though it has been 4,000 years since King Chieh (the last king of the legendary Xia dynasty [21st-16th century BC]) and King Chou (the last king of the Shang or Yin dynasty [16th century-1066 BC]) tyrannically governed the people, they are still held up to be symbols of immorality and corruption, thus illustrating people's hatred for vice.

Confucius had over 3,000 disciples, but only Yen Hui sustained complete virtue for three months. Other disciples could only manage to sustain complete virtue for one month, and some only for one day. The fact that only 72 disciples were willing to follow Confucius with their hearts illustrates the incomparable selfishness of people.

King Wen, the founder of the Zhou dynasty (1066-221 BC),

lived by a strict moral code and died at the age of 100, but his moral influence did not spread out into the world. King Wu (son of King Wen) and the Duke of Zhou (younger brother of King Wu) succeeded King Wen's moral establishments and greatly influenced people throughout their kingdom. Nevertheless, Kwan Shu and Chai Shu rebelled against their brother, the Duke of Zhou demonstrating that there is truly nothing comparable to the iniquities of people.

6) A Mind Set to Deceive the World Is Always Hidden

People's inherent nature can be likened to that of King Yao and King Shun; however, people's knowledge and conduct cannot. When people's ears, eyes, nose, and mouth possess an affinity for virtue, their minds are akin to Yao's and Shun's. When people's Lungs, Spleen, Liver and Kidneys detest vice, their minds are akin to Yao's and Shun's. However, there are deceptive tendencies hidden in the jaw, chest, waist, and abdomen. So, people may become as wise as Yao and Shun only after preserving their true mind and cultivating their true nature. There are also deceptive tendencies hidden in the head, shoulders, waist and hips. So people can only conduct themselves like Yao and Shun after they learn to regulate themselves and establish proper values.

7) A Selfish Mind that Is Arrogant, Pretentious, Cruel, and Boastful Throws away Wisdom

It is evident that people's ears, eyes, nose, and mouth have an affinity for virtue, since people tend to agree upon what is righteous even though they have different backgrounds. In reality, people's affinity for virtue is extremely impartial. It contains no selfish motives. The reason that the Lungs, Spleen, Liver and Kidneys dislike vice is that although people may be in a close relationship, they are still looking to benefit themselves in their own ways. The reality of people's dislike for vices is extremely impartial and contains no selfish motives.

People prefer virtue to vice, but people quickly lose their natural wisdom cultivated and polished in the jaw, chest, navel and abdomen and act improperly because the selfish minds of arrogance, pretentiousness, cruelty and boasting appear. Virtuous conduct firmly resides in the head, shoulders, waist and hips. Yet when the greedy minds of depriving, extravagance, indolence and pilfering appear, they eliminate noble actions and lead people astray. It is, therefore, necessary to eliminate the selfish and greedy minds through conscientious effort.

8) The *Tao* and Virtue Originate from Self-realization and One's Occupation

Tao and virtue originate from self-realization and one's occupation. Heaven made this possible for all people. The origin of *tao* resides in one's daily life and profession, such as scholar, farmer, craftsman, and merchant, as well as the places where one's life and profession take place such as fields, houses, states and countries. The source of virtue is in self-realization which gives rise to all virtuous conduct, such as benevolence, righteousness, propriety, wisdom, loyalty, devotion friendship, and fraternal love.

Only when one has a great deal more wisdom than others, can one truly teach others. Only when one's means of livelihood is honest, can one establish merit. No matter how distinguished a person may be, if he is selfish, trivial, and cunning like Cao Cao (one of the last great generals of the Han dynasty, yet he is generally depicted as the archetypal shrewd, bold and unscrupulous villain), he cannot teach others. Even though a person's accomplishments may be renowned, if he is violent and cruel like the Emperor of Qin, the founder of the first unified Chinese empire (259-210 BC), he can receive no merit.

It is a great virtue when one can appreciate the good deeds

of others while performing good deeds oneself. It is the righteous *tao* to dislike the evil deeds of others while not performing evil deeds oneself. A person who has a virtuous mind is constantly cultivating his or her mind.

9) Preserving the Clarity of Mind Equates Rebuking the Mind

In order to preserve the clarity of one's mind it is necessary to constantly rebuke one's mind. It may seem as though the clarity and turbidity of the mind occur spontaneously, however, the mind that is rebuked is clear while the mind that is not rebuked is turbid. The reason that a horse is sharper and smarter than a cow is that a horse rebukes its mind more than a cow. The reason that a hawk is fiercer than a kite (an Asian black bird) is that the hawk rebukes its mind more than a kite. If the clarity and turbidity of the mind, and the strength and weakness of the physical body are such a way in animals then how can human beings be any different?

3. A Discourse on the Four Principles

This section will introduce certain parts of "A Discourse on the Four Principles" found in *Longevity and Life Preservation in Eastern Medicine.*

Many remarkable methods of health cultivation have been handed down from the past, but none have emphasized the particularities of individual constitutions more than SCM.

The original Sasang Theory was based on the *Four Principles* according to Mencius, which are benevolence, righteousness, propriety and wisdom. Benevolence is a feeling of empathy, sympathy or compassion for the misfortune or pain of others. Righteousness is a dislike or shame for things that are immoral or unethical. Propriety is a respect for elders or superiors and humility or modesty. Wisdom is the ability to distinguish between right and wrong. According to Mencius, these characteristics are innate human natures that are common to all people. Human beings are born with a virtuous nature and can become noble or develop into a sage by amplifying the *Four Principles.*

Expanding on Mencius' *Four Principles*, Dr. Lee Je-ma states that in order to cultivate one's character so that there are no defects or prejudices, different methods should be employed according to individual constitutions. People need to understand the particularities of their constitutions in order to supplement their weaknesses. They should also remain vigilant of erroneous behaviors and cultivate their talents and abilities.

1) A Discourse on the Four Principles of Human Beings

Taeyangin, Soyangin, Tae-eumin and *Soeumin* are the *Four Principles* of human beings. *Taeyangin* has large Lungs and a small Liver, *Soyangin* has a large Spleen and small Kidneys, *Tae-eumin* has a large Liver and small Lungs, and *Soeumin* has large Kidneys and a small Spleen.

Rudeness, superficiality, greed, and indolence are the *Four Principles* of human desire. Those who throw away propriety and do whatever pleases them are called Mean. Those who throw away wisdom and subtly try to deceive others are called Superficial. Those who are not benevolent and only want to fill their selfish desires are called Avaricious. Those who throw away righteousness and scheme only to comfort themselves are called Weak.

When benevolence, righteousness, propriety, and wisdom are fully realized, there will be a *vast flowing qi* and when rudeness, superficiality, greed, and indolence are driven out, *vast flowing Principle* will manifest.

Though sages are said to have no selfish desires, this does not mean that they have no desire itself as in Lao Tzu or

Buddha. Since sages are concerned with issues of the world, they have no time to pay attention to their selfish greed. Thus, they do not hesitate to learn or to teach others. This is the true meaning behind the unselfishness of the sage. The hearts of King Yao and King Shun do not hold even the slightest selfish desire. The hearts of Confucius and Mencius hold great concern for the world at all times.

2) Though One's Heart Loves Virtue...

Though one's heart loves virtue, if it is partial and hasty it will not be just. Though one's heart detests vices, if it is partial and hasty it will not be widely known. It is better to work with virtuous people. If not, joy, and pleasure will certainly be disturbed. If you work with wicked people, sorrow and anger will increase ever more.

3) Sorrow and Anger Generate Each Other

Sorrow and anger generate each other and joy and pleasure complement one another. If *Taeyangin's* sorrow is so extreme that it cannot be controlled, anger will spring forth. If *Soyangin's* anger is so severe that it cannot be controlled, sorrow will fill the heart. If *Soeumin's* excessive pleasure is uncontrolled, joy will become unsettled. If *Tae-eumin's* excessive joy is uncontrolled, pleasure will be unrestrained. Such a strong stirring of emotions can be compared to cutting one's intestines with a knife so that 10 years will not be enough to recover health. This will determine life and death, longevity and premature death. That is why it must never be forgotten.

4) If Sorrow, Anger, Joy, and Pleasure Manifest in an Appropriate Manner then One Is in a State of Harmony

If sorrow, anger, joy and pleasure are not stirred within, then one is in a state of equilibrium. If they manifest in an appropriate manner then one is in a state of harmony. A person who does not express sorrow, anger, joy, and pleasure, yet who is constantly vigilant of his emotions, will he not gradually become similar to a person who is in a state of equilibrium? And a person who expresses sorrow, anger, joy, and pleasure, yet reflects upon them, is he not similar to a person who is in a state of harmony?

4. A Discourse on Five Blessings

The "A Discourse on Five Blessings" explains the five things that we should value most in our lives, their individual significance, their level of importance and which one should take precedence in order for them to have meaning. Since "A Discourse on Five Blessings" is short, it is discussed in its entirety.

1) The Five Things That Are Most Joyful in Life

There are five things in life that bring the most joy; longevity, a virtuous mind, desire for reading, building a family wealth, and following through with one's plan in the world.

A virtuous mind means nothing without longevity. Reading is useless without the proper use of knowledge. Wealth cannot be gained without reading (studying). Without family support, plans will not succeed even with proper assessment and implementation.

Therefore, nothing is useful without longevity. Even a wicked person should attempt to acquire longevity. People should have virtuous minds even though they do not study or read books. People should read books even though they cannot build family wealth. People should build family wealth even though they are unable to follow through with their goals in the world.

Therefore, a person who attempts to follow through with his goals without family support is in vain. A person who is wealthy but does not read is a fool, a person who reads books without a virtuous mind is a swindler, and a person who has virtuous mind without longevity is inferior.

2) All Diseases Arise from Emotional Stress

All diseases arise from emotional stress. Scholars should eat just two meals a day and even farmers should only occasionally eat three meals per day. Regardless of the difficulties or tribulations one may face, as long as a person does not become overly emotional, he or she should be able to achieve longevity. Fortune or misfortune should befall any person who actively seeks them. And longevity or premature death should occur when they are actively sought after.

3) It Is Easy to Acquire Family Wealth but Hard to Gain Knowledge

It is easier to acquire wealth than knowledge through reading. Simple things are easy to acquire but difficult things are hard to acquire. Therefore, reading should take precedence over gathering wealth.

Wealth is acquired through diligence, an ability that everybody has. In contrast, knowledge is earned through intelligence, which is an ability possessed only by certain people with talent.

4) A Person with Talent but without Virtue Is a Narrow-minded Person

A person who has talent but is without virtue is a narrow-minded person. A narrow-minded person can be compared to a peasant.

One might ask how a diligent peasant could be compared to a narrow-minded person, just because he does not read. The answer is that a gentleman who reads a lot of books is considered to be the best, then a diligent peasant, then a scholar who is not virtuous, and finally a peasant who is lazy.

Also, one might ask of what use is longevity for the wicked person? The answer is that being able to acquire longevity even though one is wicked can be compared to being able to plow the land with the use of the strength of oxen and horses. If oxen and horses are useful then how can human beings be not useful in this world? Even oxen and horses try to live long lives, so why would human beings not wish to live long lives?

5) Children Will Die Prematurely If Medicine Is Applied Inappropriately

There are many cases of children afflicted with serious illnesses dying prematurely due to the indiscriminate use of popular medicines. Even though children have serious diseases, most of them can recover if they can avoid severe temperature changes, maintain a proper diet, and get a lot of fresh air. However, if medicines are inappropriately applied, about one half of these children could easily die. For acute illnesses, medicines can be used only after thoroughly questioning their appropriateness.

5. A Discourse on Knowledge and Conduct

Dr. Lee Je-ma's philosophy is not simply speculation. It is rather a pragmatic path and the philosophy of knowledge and conduct. The path of knowledge and conduct is discussed in all of Dr. Lee Je-ma's writings, including *Longevity and Life Preservation in Eastern Medicine.* Though the magnitude, importance and methodology of knowledge and conduct are discussed in this section, the entirety of SCM and Sasang philosophy should be seen as the culmination of Dr. Lee Je-ma's discourse on knowledge and conduct.

1) Understanding with the Mind and Performing with the Body

With what do you know? Know with the mind. With what do you act? Act with the body. One's attitude should not be debauched because knowledge will be damaged. One should not desperately chase after immediate comfort because proper conduct will be lost.

Although a person interested in debauchery has a presence of mind, it is nonetheless the same as an absence of mind. If there is an absence of mind, where can knowledge come from? A person who only focuses on immediate comfort may seem like he has a body but the body does not exist. Since there is no body where can the conduct come from? Therefore, a person who is debauched is like a fool, while a person who controls his mind calmly is a sage. A person who wants to get instant comfort is an unworthy person, while a person whose body is agile and strong is a wise man.

The way of learning is to calmly control the debauched mind. This is called sincerity. The way of speculation is to quickly and forcefully rule over the comfort seeking body. This is called respect.

2) There Are Varying Degrees of Knowledge and Conduct

There are varying degrees of knowledge. Governing a nation and creating peace in the world requires *greater knowledge*, while livelihoods such as agriculture, industry, commerce, and low ranking government offices require *lesser knowledge*. There are also varying degrees of conduct. Properly wearing one's attire and behaving properly in one's daily life is considered *greater conduct*, while carrying firewood or cultivating a farm is considered *lesser conduct*.

Both knowledge and conduct must be combined in varying degrees. If only important things are attended to and less important things ignored, then the important things will never be achieved. If only trivial matters are emphasized and important matters ignored, then even the trivial things cannot be maintained.

3) If the Golden Mean Is Achieved, All Conducts, whether Great or Small, Will Be Virtuous

If the Golden Mean is achieved, all conducts, whether great or small, will be virtuous. If the Golden Mean is not achieved, all conducts, whether great or small, are wicked.

Why is this so? If a poor person carries firewood and cultivates his farm, this represents the Golden Mean and is virtuous. But if a poor person wears the attire of the noble class and behaves like he is of the noble class, the Golden Mean is not achieved and instead it is a wicked act.

If a member of the noble class correctly wears his attire and behaves properly, he is truly performing the Golden Mean and is virtuous. However, if that person carries firewood, cultivates the farm, and is busy on the streets, the Golden Mean is not achieved and instead this behavior is considered wicked.

Therefore, even though a person is in agriculture, industry, commerce, or a low government position, as long as he does not forget the knowledge of governing the nation and making world peace, there is certainly much knowledge hidden in his heart.

And as long as a person does not forget the act of carrying firewood and cultivating his farm even though he is wearing noble attire and behaving properly, there will certainly be greater conduct hidden in his body.

Appendix 1

Theories of Constitutional Disease Syndromes

Dr. Lee Je-ma stated that human beings have different prenatal patterns that manifest as different size internal organs in each constitution.* These size differences in the organs, in turn, create physiological and pathological differences, which require varying treatment principles.

Dr. Lee Je-ma claimed, in "A Discourse on the Origin of Eastern Medicine," that Zhang Zhong-jing diagnosed the disease syndromes and pharmacology of *Soeumins* in detail, but that it was the doctors of the Song, Yuan and Ming dynasties who developed these theories to their completion. Zhang Zhong-jing also partially diagnosed the disease syndromes and pharmacology of *Soyangins*, and once again, the doctors of the Song, Yuan and Ming dynasties developed these theories to near completion. The disease syndromes and pharmacology of *Tae-eumins* were scantily diagnosed by Zhang Zhong-jing and these theories were developed to about one-half of their completion by the later doctors. Zhu Zhen-heng (1281-1358 AD) captured only a shadow of the disease syndromes and pharmacology of *Taeyangins*, which are briefly mentioned in the Materia Medica.

Dr. Lee Je-ma related the Sasang constitutions to Zhang Zhong-jing's Theory of Six Channels (*Shanghanlun*) in this way: He said that all three *yin* Syndromes are *Soeumin* syndromes, all of the *shaoyang* syndromes are *Soyangin* syndromes, and the *taiyang* and *yangming* syndromes are predominantly syndromes of *Soeumins*. However, they relate to *Soyangins* and *Tae-eumins* as well. This is summarized in the following table. (p. 160)

There are a few things that need to be taken into consideration in order to understand the theory of Sasang disease syndromes. First, the Heart, Lungs, Spleen, Liver and Kidneys should be understood in a different light from traditional Syndrome Medicine's concepts of the organs. Secondly, the Sasang energetic theories of *yin-yang*, Upper-Lower and Ascending-Descending must be applied when observing and explaining the human body, rather than the cyclical Five

* verifiable how? Living: full body scans; Dead: autopsy. Any such study?

Comparison of Six Channel Syndromes and Sasang Constitutions

Six Channel Syndromes	*Soeumin*	*Soyangin*	*Tae-eumin*	*Taeyangin*
Taiyang Syndromes	O	O	O	O
Yangming Syndromes	O	O	O	O
Shaoyang Syndromes		X		
Taiyin Syndromes	X			
Shaoyin Syndromes	X			
Jueyin Syndromes	X			

O: Related Syndrome
X: Syndrome related to a specific constitution

Element Theory. Thirdly, the Exterior-Interior and Heat-Cold syndromes of the Eight Principles should be understood in terms of the system of constitutional syndrome differentiation that explains the tangible and intangible phenomena of the *yin-yang* variance, with the typical differences of the individual as the premise. Lastly, the concepts of Exterior *yin*, Interior *yang*, Clear *yang* and so forth must be understood in terms of Righteous *qi* rather than Pathogenic *qi*.

Prior to delving into an explanation of each Sasang constitutional disease syndrome, I will first classify the contents of the constitutional syndromes into simple terms, as is done in the following table. Then I will summarize the particular characteristics of the constitutional disease syndromes and their appropriate treatment methods (Note: A complete list of herbal formulas for the following syndromes can be found in Appendix 4.).

Table of Sasang Constitutional Disease Syndromes

		Soeumin	*Soyangin*	*Tae-eumin*	*Taeyangin*
Exterior Disease	Mild	Manic Syndrome	Soyang Wind Injury Syndrome	Taeyang Extreme Cold Syndrome	*Hae Yuk* Syndrome
	Severe	Yang Collapse Syndrome	Yin Collapse Syndrome	Esophagus Cold Syndrome	
Interior Disease	Mild	Tae-eum Syndrome	Chest Heat Syndrome	Liver Heat Syndrome	*Yul Gyuk* Syndrome
	Severe	Soeum Syndrome	Yin Deficiency Tidal Fever Syndrome	Dry-Heat Syndrome	

(1) *Soeumin* Disease Syndromes

Soeumin disease syndromes are classified into two main groups: *Exterior Febrile Disease induced from the Kidney affected by Heat* and *Interior Cold Disease induced from the Stomach affected by Cold.*

When the Kidney *yin* becomes exuberant due to the large Kidneys, the excess cold that is created hinders the Kidney *yang* from ascending and makes it stagnant causing the *Exterior Febrile Disease induced from the Kidney affected by Heat*. This disease is classified into *Manic Syndrome* and *Yang Collapse Syndrome* and each of these syndromes are further divided into initial, middle and terminal stages. The initial stage of *Manic Syndrome* has symptoms of restlessness and irritability that occur when a Taiyang exterior syndrome is unresolved. In the middle stage, the constipation related to the *Yangming Fu Syndrome* develops. The terminal stage manifests with a tidal fever, delirious speech, shortness of breath, and a fixed gaze that occur in the *Yangming Syndrome.*

The initial stage of *Yang Collapse Syndrome* presents with the chills, fever, and spontaneous sweating of *Taiyang Syndrome*. The middle stage includes a high fever without chills and spontaneous sweating that are related to the *Yangming Syndrome*. The terminal stage manifests with the high fever and profuse sweating also of the *Yangming Syndrome. Manic Syndrome* manifests with a fever and an absence of sweating while *Yang Collapse Syndrome* has a fever with spontaneous sweating. Thus *Yang Collapse Syndrome* is more severe than *Manic Syndrome*.

Sweating is seen as dangerous in *Soeumins* because this constitution has a weakness in their ascending energy and in their Spleen, which predisposes them to *yang* deficiency. Thus sweating in *Soeumins* indicates a further weakening of the *yang* and when the sweating continues, the *yang* will likely collapse. Therefore, in both *Manic Syndrome* and *Yang Collapse Syndrome* the basic treatment focuses on raising the *yang* energy that is not ascending.

An absence of sweating in *Manic Syndrome* indicates the existence of *yang qi.* Because this is a situation in which there is a disharmony between only the *ying* (Nutritive) and the *wei* (Protective), the treatment principle is to harmonize the *ying* and *wei.* The sweating present in *Yang Collapse Syndrome* is the exterior leakage of body fluids. Thus the fundamental treatment is the application of the *Raise the yang and Augment the qi* method in order to raise the *yang qi.*

In the exterior disease of *Soeumins*, *Blood Stagnation in the Lower Burner Syndrome* manifests with mania due to heat stagnating in the Urinary Bladder from an unresolved *Taiyang* Syndrome or an improper treatment. This is called *Kidney yang Distressed by Heat.* The treatment involves using Ligusticum and Cinnamon Decoction (*Chunkoongkaeji tang*), Astragalus and Cinnamon Decoction (*Hwangkikaeji tang*) and Eight Noble Ingredient Decoction (*Palmulkeunja tang*) to raise the stagnant *yang qi.*

Lower Abdominal Fullness Syndrome also known as *Large Intestine Aversion to Cold Syndrome* is caused by a chronic unresolved Exterior Syndrome combined with an Interior Syndrome. It should first be harmonized with the formulas Agastache Powder to Rectify the *qi* (*Kwakhyangchungki san*) or Nourish the Stomach Decoction with Cyperus and Cardamon (*Hyangsayangwi tang*) after which the *yang qi* should be raised. If Exterior Heat is surrounding the Interior Cold, croton (ba dou) should be used to cause diarrhea and then a harmonizing treatment should be applied.

In contrast, *Interior Cold Disease induced from the Stomach affected by Cold* is distinguished by the severity of the *yin qi. Soeumins*' particular attribute of having a small Spleen results in a constant lack of Spleen *yang* that causes a stagnation of *yin* and a lack of rising *yang.* The basic symptoms are abdominal pain and diarrhea and the disease is divided into *Tae-eum* or *Soeum Syndromes. Tae-eum Syndrome* has abdominal pain and diarrhea with an absence of thirst, while *Soeum Syndrome* has abdominal pain and diarrhea with thirst. Therefore, the existence or absence of irritability, appetite and thirst are the important indices for differentiating between these two syndromes.

The diarrhea of *Tae-eum Syndrome* indicates that the warm *qi* of the Stomach is dispelling the cold *qi* of the Large Intestine, while the diarrhea of *Soeum Syndrome* indicates that the cold *qi* of the Large Intestine is putting pressure on the warm *qi* of the Stomach. *Tae-eum Syndrome* is a mild syndrome, while *Soeum Syndrome* is a severe, rebellious syndrome that is a combination of both an exterior and an interior disease. The treatment principle for both of these syndromes is to descend the excessive *yin qi* that is stagnant. In *Tae-eum Syndrome*, since the warm *qi* is expelling the cold *qi*, the proper treatment method augments the warm *qi* while descending the Internal *yin* (cold). This is a method to warm the Stomach and descend the *yin.* Because *Soeum Syndrome* is a state in which the Righteous *qi* is weakened allowing a deeper region to be affected, the treatment method used strengthens the Spleen and descends the *yin.* Other syndromes, such as *Jang Kwal (Visceral Shock) Syndrome* or *Exuberance of Yin Dispelling Yang Syndrome*, are similar to the *Soeum Syndrome*, as are their treatment methods. Nevertheless, all of these syndromes should be treated in their initial stages.

As mentioned above, *Soeumins*' overall center of strength lies in the lower part of their bodies (Lower Burner) so they are predisposed to an excess of *yin.* For this reason, the ascending-descending treatment concept should be applied based on the principle of *yang qi Maintaining Life.* The treatment for the Exterior Syndrome focuses on transforming the *yin qi* that exists due to the large Kidneys into *yang* through the *Raise the yang and Augment the qi* method. Interior Syndrome treatment focuses on releasing excessive *yin qi* through the method of *Descending the Interior yin.*

(2) *Soyangin* Disease Syndromes

Soyangins have a large Spleen and small Kidneys. Their syndromes are divided into *Exterior Cold Disease induced from the Spleen affected by Cold* and *Interior Febrile Disease induced from the Stomach affected by Heat.*

Exterior Cold Disease induced from the Spleen affected by Cold occurs when the *yin qi* cannot descend due to a build up of pressure by the excessive *yang qi* of the Spleen. Because *Soyangins*' Spleens are large, they have strong *yang* energy. For the sake of convenience, Spleen *yin* is referred to as Exterior *yin.* The exterior disease is differentiated into *Soyang Wind Injury* and *Yin Collapse* depending on the severity of the stagnation of the Exterior *yin.*

In *Soyang Wind Injury*, pathogenic heat causes the *yin qi* of the Kidneys to sink and the *yin qi* of the Spleen to become stagnant. The stagnant Spleen *yin qi* cannot descend to the Kidneys, so it gathers between the shoulders and upper back. This manifests with chills and fever, body aches, an absence of sweating, irritability, and a superficial and tight pulse. Other symptoms such as a bitter taste in the mouth, dry throat, dizziness, tinnitus, alternating chills and fever, and vomiting are included in this category.

If *Soyang Wind Injury* goes unresolved for many days, this not only prevents the Exterior *yin* from descending, it also prevents the Interior *yang* from ascending and *Chest Knotting Syndrome* develops. Here, there are symptoms of epigastric fullness and tightness with nausea, shortness of breath, and in severe cases other symptoms, such as delirious speech, constipation and mania appear. Therefore, *Soyang Wind Injury* should be treated by clearing the Interior Heat and descending the Exterior *yin* to prevent *Chest Knotting Syndrome.* Since *Chest Knotting Syndrome* is a combination of an Interior and Exterior Syndromes, the more urgent symptoms should be treated first.

The typical symptom of *Yin Collapse Syndrome* is diarrhea. This syndrome occurs due to a rebellious upward flow of the *yin qi*, which is supposed to descend. For *Yin Collapse* with symptoms of fever, headache, and diarrhea, Polyporus and Plantain Decoction (*Juhryungchajunja tang*) and Sedate the White Powder with Schizonepeta and Sileris (*Hyungbangsabaek san*) should be given. For *Yin Collapse* with a cold body, abdominal pain, and diarrhea, Talcum and Sophora Decoction (*Hwalsukkosam tang*) and Rehmannia Decoction with Schizonepeta and Sileris (*Hyungbangjihwang tang*) can be prescribed. *Soyang Wind Injury* is a mild disease, while *Yin Collapse Syndrome* is more severe. *Chest Knotting Syndrome* is a disharmonious syndrome of both the Exterior and the Interior.

The *Interior Febrile Disease induced from the Stomach affected by Heat* that affects *Soyangins* is caused by the inability of the clear *yang* (Interior *yang*) to ascend. This Interior Yang that is unable to ascend is called the "Diminished *yang*" or "Fire." Disease occurs from the *Yin* Deficiency resulting from the small Kidneys compounded by an inability of the clear *yang* or the *yuan qi* (Source *qi*) to reach the head and four extremities smoothly. Instead, it transforms into pathogenic heat. This interior disease is divided into *Chest Heat Syndrome* and *Yin Deficiency Tidal Fever Syndrome.*

Chest Heat Syndrome occurs due to an inability of the Interior *yang* to ascend and instead transforming into pathogenic heat. Its main symptom is constipation, which can present with other symptoms of Heat and Fire such as *Upper and Middle Wasting and Thirsting Syndromes (diabetes)*, night sweats, carbuncles on the back, furuncles on the head, swelling of the lips, throat diseases, *yang* toxins with rashes, erysipelas, jaundice and diseases of ears, eyes, mouth, nose, and teeth. The severity of the disease is determined by the degree of constipation. If a *Soyangin* cannot have a bowel movement for several days, it indicates that the *yang* toxins have become severe. This is called *Interior Heat Constipation* and needs to be treated immediately with White Tiger Decoction with Rehmannia (*Jihwangbaekho tang*) to open the blockage.

The method to release the stagnant Fire that is in the middle regions of *Soyangins*' bodies is called *Clearing Heat and Sedating Fire*. It is namely a method to ascend the clear *yang*. The formula Cool the Diaphragm and Disperse the Fire Decoction (*Yanggyuksanhwa tang*) is most frequently prescribed for this purpose.

The syndrome of *Yin Deficiency Tidal Fever* is caused by an inability of the Interior *yang* to ascend and the Exterior *yin* to descend. The Interior *yang* cannot ascend because of the *Soyangin's* particular characteristic of having small Kidneys. The inability of the Interior *yang* to ascend brings about symptoms of *yin* deficiency with false heat such as afternoon fever, thirst, upper back chills, and nausea. Additional symptoms include lower *Wasting and Thirsting Syndrome*, stroke and vomiting blood. This syndrome is treated with the method of *Tonifying the yin and Descending the Fire* in order to raise the clear *yang*.

In general, most of the energetic strength of *Soyangins* is situated in the upper region of their bodies. This implies that their bodies are *yang* in nature and can easily manifest symptoms of Heat. Thus the ascending-descending concept is applied based on the principle of *yin qi Maintaining Life*. *Soeumin* diseases are generally due to cold while *Soyangin* diseases are generally caused by Heat. The treatment of *soyang Exterior Syndrome* is to descend the Exterior *yin* that is stagnant because of the large Spleen. Meanwhile, the treatment of *soyang Interior Syndrome* is to raise the Interior *yang* (clear *yang*) in order to clear the Heat caused by the small Kidneys.

(3) *Tae-eumin* Disease Syndromes

Tae-eumins have a large Liver and small Lungs. Their syndromes are generally divided into *Exterior Cold Disease induced from the Esophagus affected by Cold* and *Interior Febrile Disease induced from the Liver affected by Heat.*

Exterior Cold Disease induced from the Esophagus affected by Cold is caused by the particular characteristic of *Tae-eumins* having small Lungs. This results in an overall lack of energy spreading out to the exterior caused by the insufficient rising power of the esophagus, its *fu* organ (paired organ), and the insufficient dispersing *qi* of the Lungs. This disease is principally divided into *Taeyang Extreme Cold Syndrome* and *Esophagus Cold Syndrome.*

When the symptoms of headache, fever, pain in the waist and joints, chills, absence of sweating and cough occur in *Taiyang shang hàn* (Injury due to Cold), it is called *Lumbar Vertebra Exterior Disease* and belongs to the category of *Taeyang Extreme Cold Syndrome.* This occurs due to a disharmony of Ying-Blood. Promoting sweating to support the dispersing *qi* can resolve this problem. This is done using the formula Ephedra Decoction to Release the Exterior (*Mahwangbalpyo tang*). *Taeyang Extreme Cold Syndrome* occurs when anxiety weakens the Esophagus. The Cold pathogen takes advantage of the situation and invades the weakened exterior. This pits the Righteous *qi* and the pathogenic *qi* against each other. Under these circumstances there will be alternating chills and fever with sweating that will repeat for several days. In order to properly treat this syndrome, the severity of the disease must be determined by the presence and the extent of the patient's sweating or the lack of sweating as a gauge. Sweating is induced with Bear Gall Bladder Powder (*Woongdam san*) or Greater Cold Lesser Heat Decoction (*Handayulso tang*) depending on the severity of the syndrome.

Exophagus Cold Syndrome is a Dry Syndrome caused by *Tae-eumins*' characteristic lack of dispersing *qi*. The symptoms include food stagnation with fullness, weakness in the legs, jaundice, spermatorrhea due to overstrain, and cough. For these symptoms, dryness is cleared with the Sweating and Moistening methods using *Tae-eum* Regulate the Stomach Decoction (*Tae-eumjowyi tang*) and Regulate the Stomach and Raise the Clear Decoction (*Jowyiseungki tang*). Accordingly, herbs that promote sweating in order to release the pathogenic factor or moisten to support the dispersing *qi* of the Lungs are used in the treatment of the *Exterior Cold Disease induced from the Esophagus affected by Cold.*

On the other hand, the *Interior Febrile Disease induced from the Liver affected by Heat* is a Heat Syndrome caused by the Tae-eumin*'s* characteristic large Liver. The large Liver creates strong gathering *qi* that prevents energy from dispersing and causes heat stagnation inside the body. This disease is mainly divided into the *Liver Heat Syndrome* and the *Dry-Heat Syndrome*.

Liver Heat Syndrome occurs due to "unrestrained pleasure and excessive desire," which cause severe Liver Heat and Lung Dryness. Included in this category are the *Yangming Channel* and *Yangming Fu Syndromes*, in which fever is the main symptom, as well as the *Shang Han Yang Toxin* or *Warm Disease. Wasting and Thirsting Syndrome* with copious urination, and other symptoms such as gangrenous blotches on the fingers, and spermatorrhea due to overstrain also belong to this syndrome, as do symptoms of deafness, visual difficulty, weakness in the legs and low back pain caused by the exhaustion of *yin* and blood. Greater Heat and Lesser Cold Decoction (*Yuldahanso tang*) is the basic formula used to clear the dry heat. Release the Muscle Layer Decoction with Kudzu (*Kalkeunhaegi tang*), Clear the Lung and Sedate the Liver Decoction (*Chungpaesakan tang*), and Lotus Seed Decoction to Clear the Heart (*Chungshimyunja tang*) can be used according to the presentation of the disease pattern.

Dry-Heat Syndrome occurs from an excess of Liver Heat causing stagnant heat in the Small Intestine, which is the Fu or paired organ of the Liver. This syndrome manifests the high fever of epidemic febrile diseases or it may present as a high fever with severe chills, constipation and urinary blockage, or fever and swelling with redness on the head, face and neck. These symptoms occur when the disease is severe. Therefore formulas such as Raise the *qi* Decoction with Kudzu (*Kalkeunseungki tang*) and Gleditsia and Rhubarb Decoction (*Jokakdaehwang tang*) should be taken immediately to promote a bowel movement that will release the Liver Heat.

In the cases mentioned above, both the Exterior and Interior Syndromes are *Dry Syndromes*. This concept of dryness is different from the idea of dryness stemming from Blood and Y*in* Deficiency held by Syndrome Medicine. The dryness of the Exterior Syndrome arises from the lack of dispersing *qi* that occurs because of the small Lungs. This is known as *Esophagus Cold* in contrast to *Liver Heat* and is released by sweating. The dryness of the Interior Syndrome is a result of stagnant heat in the interior caused by excessive gathering *qi* and is released mainly through promoting bowel movements. If the dryness is severe, herbs that nourish the blood and moisten dryness are added to both the Exterior and Interior Diseases.

(4) *Taeyangin* Disease Syndromes

Taeyangins have large Lungs and a small Liver. Their corresponding syndromes are divided into *Lumbar Vertebrae Disease induced by Exopathogen* and *Small Intestine Disease induced by Endopathogen.*

Lumbar Vertebrae Disease induced by Exopathogen is commonly called *hae yuk*. This disease presents in the waist region due to the strong dispersing *qi* of the Lungs and the weak gathering *qi* of the Liver, which create a strong upper body and a weak waist and lower body region. The waist, which is the region of the Liver, is easily attacked by external *yang* pathogens. Here the upper body is completely healthy but the lower body is weak, which causes walking difficulties. Even though there is no pain, paralysis or atrophy, the lower extremities are weak. It is a state that is "neither weak nor strong, neither cold nor hot." To treat this problem, deep sadness must be regulated and anger should be avoided in order to maintain a clear mind and settle the emotions. Together with mental control, Strengthen the Spine Decoction with Acanthopanax (*Ogapijangchuk tang*) can be used.

Small Intestine Disease induced by Endopathogen manifests with *yul gyuk* or dysphagia. The Lungs and Liver are the gateways for the gathering and dispersing of *qi* and fluids. They alternately carry out these functions. In *Taeyangins*, the Small Intestine, the *fu* organ of the Liver, is too weak to gather the cool *yin qi* from the *qi* and Fluids. By contrast, the warm dispersing *qi* of the Esophagus, the *fu* organ of the Lungs, is stronger. Therefore, when the Esophagus is in a state of dryness, the dispersing *qi* is excessive, while the gathering *qi* of the

Lower-Middle Burner is weak. The outcome is that food cannot be ingested and is instead vomited. This is known as *yul gyuk* or dysphagia. *Yul gyuk* will manifest with vomiting or a sensation that there is a blockage when food passes through the esophagus into the stomach. These symptoms are indicative of a severe disease in *Taeyangins*. To treat this disease, *Taeyangins* must control their anger and avoid eating greasy foods. They should also use Plant the Intestine Decoction with Actinidia (*Mihudengshikchang tang*).

Disease syndromes of *Taeyangins* are caused by their inherent energetic structure. They have a strong ascending and dispersing energy and a weak descending and gathering energy. Therefore, the ascending energy needs to be pulled down and gathered. Good urination indicates a healthy state. But if the energy rises even slightly, a symptom, such as foaming in the mouth, appears that must be treated immediately. Controlling anger is the most important factor in pulling down the rising energy. If *Taeyangins* are frequently angered, the rising energy becomes even stronger. Thus prior to prescribing herbal medicine, *Taeyangins* have to be in control of their deep sorrow and sudden anger. They must also avoid ingesting greasy foods. Controlling everyday emotions and regulating food intake are more important in the treatment of Taeyangin*s' diseases* than are herbal medicines. If they still get sick, then herbal prescriptions can be applied.

Dr. Lee Je-ma explained that Sasang disease syndromes are caused by variances in the *qi* that arise from the inherent differences in the sizes of the internal organs and the imbalance of the rising and descending *qi* of the nature and emotions. He introduced the Exterior, Interior, Heat, and Cold Syndromes of the Sasang constitutions and placed the Heart (which represent the *taichi*) at the center, while combining the internal organs with the principles of Exterior, Interior, Cold, and Heat. Thus he explained the speed of the movement of *yin-yang* and ascending-descending in relative terms.

Additionally, Dr. Lee Je-ma stated that, "In the past, most doctors did not know that diseases arise from an imbalance of emotions such as love, hate, desire, joy, anger, sorrow, and pleasure. Instead, they thought that diseases only developed out of injury to the Spleen and Stomach from food, or invasion of climatic factors such as wind, cold, heat and dampness." Thus, he emphasized the imbalance in one's nature and emotions as the main cause of disease. In the disease syndrome theory of the Sasang constitutions, he further stated that an imbalance of the nature and emotions of the individual constitutions will cause disease, and emphasized regulating nature and emotions more than herbal prescriptions for severe and critical conditions.

Dr. Lee Je-ma also discussed the relationship between the habitual states of emotion and disease. When the "constant minds" of the Sasang constitutions worsen, mind-body diseases manifest as moderate and severe diseases. The table below summarizes mind-body disease syndromes according to the individual constitutions.

Ultimately, because of the dual nature of the Sasang Syndromes, a multi-dimensional view, from the exterior to the interior and vice versa, must be considered when applying herbal prescriptions. This is the spirit of the application of Sasang constitutional disease syndrome differentiation. It is a method to balance one's nature and emotions from the dimension of regulating and balancing the Righteous *qi* of the body instead of tonifying and sedating according to strengths of the pathogenic *qi* and the righteous *qi*.

Mind-Body Disease Syndromes of Sasang Constitutions

Body Type	Constant Mind	Healthy State	Mild Disease	Worsening of Constant Mind	Imbalance of Emotions	Severe Disease
Taeyang	urgency	good urination	foam in the mouth	constipation for 8-9 days is not serious	extreme anger	dysphagia "cool air flowing in Esophagus"
Soyang	anxiety	good bowel movement	constipation	fear forgetfulness	stirring of sorrow	Constipation "extreme heat in chest"
Taeum	fear	sweating	diarrhea/ closing of pores	severe palpitation	unrestrained pleasure	Dysentery "clogging up Small Intestine"
Soeum	nervous-ness	good digestion	spontaneous sweating/ constant diarrhea	throat disease is mild	unstable joy	constant diarrhea "lower abdomen ice cold"

Appendix 2

The Sasang System of Dr. Lee Je-ma

The chapters preceding the appendices of this book used various topics to explain Sasang constitutions and Sasang Constitutional Medicine. As a result, each topic has been explained to some extent, but the explanations were not sufficient to describe the entirety of Dr. Lee Je-ma's philosophy. Therefore, I would like to try to summarize Dr. Lee Je-ma's entire Sasang philosophy.

(1) Ontology of the Four-Element Structure

Dr. Lee Je-ma considered the main ideas of Sasang philosophy to be "activity, mind, body, and matter." These basic units of Sasang philosophy simultaneously explain the constituents of the universe and the elements of birth, growth and change as they are found in the interpretation of the second phrase in the first chapter of the *Doctrine of the Mean*. Here it states, "Equilibrium is the foundation of all things and phenomena in the world, and harmony is their universal path. Therefore, when a state of total equilibrium and harmony manifests, proper order will be established, and all things will be nourished and will flourish."

In the chapter "Caution on Insincerity" in *Manuscript of Science*, Dr. Lee Je-ma states that the mind is *taichi*, the mind and body are the Two Modes (*yin* and *yang*), and activity, mind, body and matter are Sasang (*taeyang*, *soyang*, *tae-eum*, and *soeum*). He makes these associations in order to explain his ontological view. The *I Ching* explains the universal creative principle and differentiation processes by illustrating how the *taichi* generates the Two Modes, the Two Modes generate the Sasang, and the Sasang generates the Eight Trigrams. Fortune, misfortune, matter, and phenomena are established at the level of the Eight Trigrams. The Sasang is merely the stage between the Two Modes and the Eight Trigrams. Dr. Lee Je-ma, however, described the Sasang as a substantial concept with no further differentiation. He believed the Sasang to be the four great formative elements of the universe and viewed the Eight Trigrams as merely the dual aspects of the Sasang. Accordingly, activity, mind, body and matter are inductively used to explain all things and phenomena and this explanatory relationship forms a complex four-element structure when used to describe the phenomena of the universe, society, and the human body.

The four-element structure of the universe is said to be heaven, human, nature, and order. The constituents of social phenomena are said to be benevolence, righteousness, propriety, and wisdom (activity); loyalty, filial piety, friendship, and fraternal love (mind); the scholar, the farmer, the craftsman, and the merchant (body); as well as fields, houses, states, and countries (matter). Social phenomena are described as universal brotherhood (activity); the befriending and living of ten thousand things (matter); the gathering and communing of people from all directions (mind); and the harmonious utilization of a variety of craftsmen (body).

To explain anatomy and physiology, the four element structure of the human body was differentiated into ears, eyes, nose, and mouth (activity); Lungs, Spleen, Liver, and Kidneys (mind); head, shoulders, waist and hips (body); and jaw, chest, navel, and abdomen (matter). Constitutions were explained in the same fashion. *Taeyangins* (activity) have large Lungs and a small Liver, *Soyangins* (mind) have a large Spleen and small Kidneys, *Soeumins* (body) have large Kidneys and a small Spleen and *Tae-eumins* (matter) have a large Liver and small Lungs. These relationships classify all universal phenomena and matter, including the human body, into activity, mind, body, and matter.

However, the substantial aspects of activity, mind, body, and matter cannot exist independently. They must undergo an internal developmental process of the "mind" of *taichi* and the "mind and body" of the Two Modes (*yin* and *yang*), prior to their appearance as the activity, mind, body and matter of the Sasang. This is where the dual aspects of nature and desire exist.

> Matter is a home for the body, the body is a residence for the mind and the mind houses activity. Matter stops, the body acts, the mind thinks and activity decides. Ten thousand things live, ten thousand bodies befriend one another, ten thousand minds gather, and ten thousand activities unfold.

Ten thousand activities are grand, a single mind is small, a single body is close by, and all things in nature are distant.

Facial expression, speech, vision, and hearing are the *Four Principles* of activity. Differentiating, thinking, asking, and learning are the *Four Principles* of the mind. Bending, releasing, gathering and extending are the *Four Principles* of the body. Willpower, courage, contemplation, and intention are the *Four Principles* of matter.

Manuscript of Science, "Summary of Confucianism" "Activity and Matter"

Taichi is the mind. Mind and body are the Two Modes. Sasang is activity, mind, body, and matter. The Eight Trigrams are the beginning and end of activity, the root and branch of matter, the moderation and urgency of the mind, and the congenital and acquired aspects of the body.

The body has two applications, sincerity of the body and respect of the body. The mind also has two applications, the righteous mind and the selfish mind. The sincerity and respect of the body are the congenital and acquired aspects of the body. Sincerity arises from the Heaven trigram and respect arises from the Earth trigram. The righteousness and selfishness of the mind are the left and right aspects of the mind. The righteous mind arises from the Fire trigram while the selfish mind arises from the Water trigram.

Manuscript of Science, "Caution on Insincerity" "Wind Caution"

There are four environmental frames: locality, human relationships, social relationships, and the times of heaven. There are four human relationships: living quarters, clanships, social acquaintances, and appointed roles.

The ears, eyes, nose, and mouth perceive heaven. The Lungs, Spleen, Liver and Kidneys are established in humans. The jaw, chest, navel, and abdomen display wisdom. The head, shoulders, waist and hips administer conduct.

Longevity and Life Preservation in Eastern Medicine,
"A Discourse on Nature and Order"

As brethren of the world, people with virtue will receive a great deal of support while those who are selfish will receive little support. The mind of a superficial person is always anxious and worried.

In befriending and living of ten thousand things, a person who is cautious and kind-hearted will prosper while a person who is cruel and cold-hearted will perish. The heart of the greedy person is always extremely fearful.

People gather and commune from all directions. People who are prudent and meticulous will succeed while those who act without formality will be unable to associate with others. The heart of a weak person is always angry.

When utilizing a variety of artisans, employ the one with a sense of humility and not the one who steals and is lazy since he will not be able to perform his duties. The heart of a mean person always enjoys recreational activities.

Manuscript of Science, "Summary of Confucianism"

(2) Lee Je-ma's View on Humanity

Dr. Lee Je-ma observed the human body in terms of the four-element structure and divided it into ears-eyes-nose-mouth, Lungs-Spleen-Liver- Kidneys, jaw-chest-navel-abdomen, and head-shoulders-waist-hips. He then explained these four groups of structures by correlating them to heaven, human, knowledge, and conduct. In other words, he stated that the ears, eyes, nose, and mouth perceive heaven; the Lungs, Spleen, Liver, and Kidneys are established in humans; the jaw, chest, navel, and abdomen display knowledge; and head, shoulders, waist, and hips administer conduct. Thus, through the synthesis of the physiological functions, ethical talents, and actual practices, Dr. Lee Je-ma considered the human body to be the unity of the four-element structure that embraces both the physical and metaphysical realms.

Dr. Lee Je-ma described King Yao and King Shun as ideal figures of humanity, and stated that the highest goal of human beings is to become sages like these two kings. He presented the viewpoint of both equality and the difference between sages and ordinary people, where the sage is the ideal figure and the ordinary person aspires to become the ideal. He stressed that the original nature of the sage is the same as that of an ordinary person because the strengths and weaknesses of the internal organs are innately identical. The eyes, ears, nose, and mouth carry the same affinity for virtue and the Lungs, Spleen, Liver, and Kidneys hold the same dislike for evil. Thus all people equally share the *Four Principles* and no differences exist in the attributes of their natural dispositions.

Sages and ordinary people differ, however, in the vices of the jaw, chest, navel, and abdomen and the idleness of the head, shoulders, waist, and hips because the innate nature of ordinary people is hidden by selfishness and greed so that they cannot be impartial. Therefore, the factor that distinguishes the sage from the ordinary person is the clarity or turbidity of the mind, which manifests as rudeness, superficiality, greed, and indolence depending upon the degree of selfishness. The difference between the sage and the ordinary person is not related to the nature of the organs nor is it related to talent, rather it stems from a fault of the mind. Dr. Lee Je-ma added that when the *qi* of the four organs (benevolence, righteousness, propriety, and wisdom) is fully developed, the *vast flowing qi* emerges, and when the mental desires (rudeness, superficiality, greed, and indolence) are identified, the *vast flowing principle* emerges. The clarity and turbidity of the mind and the strength and weakness of the body depend upon the rebuking of the mind and the body. In this we see that the primary requisite to becoming a sage boils down to proper knowledge and conduct.

These thoughts of Dr. Lee Je-ma's express how the ordinary people can become sages if they do their best to eliminate selfish greed and recover their true nature. The ears, eyes, nose, and mouth's affinity for virtue and the Lungs, Spleen, Liver, and Kidneys' dislike for vices can lead an individual to become like King Yao and King Shun. However, the vices of the jaw, chest, navel, and abdomen, and the idleness of the head, shoulders, waist, and hips can prevent one from becoming like Yao and Shun. Having an affinity for virtue and distaste for vice is the state of the true mind (*tao*) that creates a foundation for all possibilities. Vices and idleness, on the other hand, are selfish desires that become the target of self-regulation. With this in mind, Dr. Lee Je-ma stated that one could attain the knowledge and conduct of a sage only after preserving the clarity of mind, nurturing one's nature, cultivating one's body and establishing heavenly order. The accumulation of such knowledge and conduct become the morals and virtues that form the benevolent nature of a sage. This demonstrates the path of spiritual evolution for all people regardless of position. It also demonstrates a positive view of human beings.

As a result, Dr. Lee Je-ma viewed sages such as King Yao and King Shun to be ideal human beings. He also categorized humans into four levels, the scholar, the wise, the fool, and the unworthy, stating that anyone could become a sage with enough effort. His view presented the sage as a positive and self-controlled human being who emphasizes rebuking the mind and the body. He also identified the sage as a practical person of high moral code who could be seen as a person who possesses knowledge of common wisdom and who exhibits proper conduct in his livelihood.

> The ears, eyes, nose, and mouth perceive heaven. The Lungs, Spleen, Liver and Kidneys are established in humans. The jaw, chest, navel, and abdomen display knowledge. The head, shoulders, waist, and hips administer conduct.
>
> Nothing is comparable to the human ears, eyes, nose and mouth's affinity for virtue, and the Lungs, Spleen, Liver and Kidneys' dislike of evil. Nothing is comparable to the vice of the human jaw, chest, navel, and abdomen, and the idleness of the human head, shoulders, waist and hips.
>
> Through the ears, eyes, nose, and mouth, everyone can become like King Yao and King Shun, but through the jaw, chest, navel, and abdomen, not everyone can spontaneously become like Yao and Shun. Through the Lungs, Spleen, Liver, and Kidneys, everyone can become like Yao and Shun, but through the head, shoulders, waist and hips, not everyone can spontaneously become like Yao and Shun.
>
> The ears, eyes, nose, and mouth correspond to Heaven, which is wise. The Lungs, Spleen, Liver and Kidneys

correspond to human beings who are benevolent. Our jaws, chests, navels, and abdomens constitute our minds, but they are not free from foolishness. Freedom from foolishness depends on us. Our heads, shoulders, waists, and hips constitute our body, but they are not free from being unworthy. Freedom from being unworthy depends on us.

Longevity and Life Preservation in Eastern Medicine,
"A Discourse on Nature and Order"

Though there are four categories of organ formations, there is one common factor to all of the categories, the transformation of the principles of nature. This is why the sage and the ordinary person are identical. Though four different classes of mind exist, there are 10,000 different levels in each class due to the magnitude of selfish desires. This is why the sage and the ordinary person are different in 10,000 ways.

Since the organs of ordinary people are identical to those of the sage, their abilities are identical. Because ordinary people have abilities identical to a sage, the claim that ordinary people lack ability arises not from their lack of ability, but is rather a shortcoming of their minds.

The *vast flowing qi* emerges from the Lungs, Spleen, Liver and Kidneys. The *vast flowing principle* emerges from the Heart. When the *qi* of the four organs (benevolence, righteousness, propriety, and wisdom) is amplified, the *vast flowing qi* emerges from those four organs. When the desires of the mind (rudeness, superficiality, greed, and indolence) are clearly distinguished, the *vast flowing principle* emerges from the Heart.

Longevity and Life Preservation in the Eastern Medicine,
"A Discourse on the Four Principles"

Having an affinity for the virtues of others while practicing virtue oneself is the virtue of the ultimate human nature. Disliking the vices of others while having no vice oneself is the way of righteous order. Accumulation of knowledge and conduct is the Tao and the virtue. Accomplishing the Tao and the virtue is the state of a benevolent sage. The Tao and the virtue are not different from knowledge and deeds. *Nature* and *order* are not different from knowledge and deeds.

In order to preserve the clarity of one's mind it is necessary to constantly rebuke one's mind. It may seem as though the clarity and turbidity of the mind occur spontaneously, however, the mind that is rebuked is clear while the mind that is not rebuked is turbid. The reason that a horse is sharper and smarter than a cow is that a horse rebukes its mind more than a cow. The reason that a hawk is fiercer and stronger than a kite (an Asian black bird) is that the hawk rebukes its mind more than a kite. If the clarity and turbidity of the mind, and the strength and weakness of the physical body are this way in animals then how can human beings be different?

Heaven created human beings and endowed them with a sense of common wisdom as part of their nature... Virtue originates from a sense of common wisdom... Heaven created human beings and endowed them with a means of livelihood which originates from heaven's order... Tao originates from the means of livelihood.

Longevity and Life Preservation in Eastern Medicine,
"A Discourse on Nature and Order"

(3) A Discourse on the Way of Knowing Others by Lee Je-ma

Dr. Lee Je-ma stated that self-cultivation (an unwavering mind) is the characteristic of a virtuous person. Specifically, this refers to maintaining balance and living in harmony with the environment. This is the middle path known as the Golden Mean. It is the same as understanding the true nature of people, in other words, knowing others. This is the starting point of the unwavering mind and self-cultivation.

Establishing sincerity of self is the prerequisite to understanding others. There exist three levels depending upon the degree to which this sincerity of self is established. The first is a situation of knowing only the superficial aspects of a person. The second occurs when one knows someone halfway. The third is gaining an understanding of the core of a person. Dr. Lee Je-ma discussed the original nature (benevolence, righteousness, propriety and wisdom) as a tangible goal of virtue when attempting to establish sincerity. He explained the desires of the mind (rudeness, superficiality, greed, and indolence) as people's most typical falsehoods that become the tangible attributes one must understand in order to know others.

Traditional Neo-Confucianism differentiates human nature and emotions by calling the *Four Principles* the "*Tao* Mind" and the seven emotions the "human mind." Dr. Lee Je-ma, on the other hand, considered sorrow, anger, joy, and pleasure together with the *Four Principles* to be human nature and distinguished this from human desire. Thus, the nature of the human beings consist of benevolence, righteousness, propriety and wisdom. Human desires consist of rudeness, superficiality, greed, and indolence, which Mencius states are the natures of the minds of the four types of people.

Dr. Lee Je-ma defined human desires by classifying the Confucian theory of "gentleman and commoner," Mencius' "biased words," "lewd words," "vulgar words," and "evasive words," and the "angry mind," "fearful mind," "pleasure-loving mind," and "anxious mind" discussed in the book, *Great Learning*, in order to explain these inclinations. In addition he claimed that one is able to gain an understanding of others through observing the sincerity of benevolence, righteousness, propriety and wisdom in immoral people and the evil desires of rudeness, superficiality, greed and indolence in good-natured people. Every person's mind contains both the mind of the gentleman and the mind of the commoner. The one that is predominant is the one that will manifest.

Meanwhile, Dr. Lee Je-ma stressed the importance of having a true understanding of a person by stating that rebellious and reckless fluctuations of sorrow, anger, joy, and pleasure are a product of insincere conduct and not having a clear understanding of others. In addition, although Dr. Lee Je-ma believed King Yao to have exemplary skills in understanding people, he stated that true understanding of others is very difficult even for King Yao, and that King Yu (known as the "Tamer of the flood," he is reputed to be the founder of

China's oldest dynasty; the Xia [21st-16th century BC]) lamented over this practice. He said that although knowing a person is extremely difficult, it must be practiced and that by using the wisdom that we all possess, there is no reason why anyone should not be able to clearly know a person. Thus Dr. Lee Je-ma emphasized the importance, as well as, the difficulty of having a true understanding of a person.

This understanding, according to Dr. Lee Je-ma's theory of the desires of the mind, points to the nature and emotion of a person who is subject to sorrow, anger, joy and pleasure. Confucius, meanwhile, explains the understanding of others through the morality (between a parent and child, a king and his subjects, siblings, and friends) of a person who is benevolent. Dr. Lee Je-ma's theory developed into the theory of the constitutional desires of the mind, which is the foundation of SCM.

> What is the reason for naming the chapter "*Self-Cultivation*?" If one likes a person even knowing his shortcomings, one can maintain a neutral position and not tilt in any way. Disliking a person yet knowing his virtue can allow one to maintain harmony with his environment. Such a person spontaneously selects the path of self-cultivation. The person who follows such a path does not have a wavering mind. If one uses all his wisdom to observe a person, there is no reason that one should not understand the person. Then what is the reason for saying that one must first be sincere before one understands others? Therefore, even if a person mobilizes all of his wisdom, a person cannot truly understand others if his sincerity is not established and, in the end, he will not know the inner mind of others or whether or not the person is dishonest.
>
> There are those who only know the superficial aspects of a person. There are those who know the core of a person. There are those who know someone halfway. There are many levels of understanding a person... Though a person may be immoral, he still has the sincerity of benevolence, righteousness, propriety, and wisdom. Though a person may be virtuous, he still has the selfish desires of rudeness,

superficiality, greed, and indolence... Gao Yao (a minister who was an expert in law and the man who enacted the punishment and prison system under King Yu) said, "You must understand a person." King Yu answered, "Yes! That is correct." This implies that one must understand others yet the understanding of others is the most difficult thing to do...Only after understanding others like King Yao, one can appreciate the wisdom and prosper. Only after one cultivates oneself like Mencius, one can dislike evil without fault.

Manuscript of Science, "Self cultivation"

Upon hearing the character of Po Yi (a sage), the greedy become pure, and the weak acquire determination. Upon hearing the character of Liu Xia Hui (also a sage), the heartless become cordial, and the mean become generous.

Mencius, Jin Xin, Part II, Verse 15

Within the mind of a person exists a gentleman's mind as well as a commoner's mind. A gentleman's mind can easily be understood but the commoner's mind is more difficult to understand. A person with a greater amount of easily comprehensible mind and a lesser amount of difficulty to comprehend the mind is called a gentleman. A person with a greater amount of an incomprehensible mind and a lesser amount of a comprehensible mind is called a commoner.

Manuscript of Science, "Caution on Insincerity" "Lake section"

King Yao controlled his sorrow, anger, joy, and pleasure so that they manifested to the proper degree since he understood how difficult it was to understand others. King Yu was able to control his sorrow, anger, joy, and pleasure so that they manifested to the proper degree because he dared not think lightly of understanding others. The sudden and reckless fluctuations of sorrow, anger, joy, and pleasure in the world arise from insincere deeds and not fully understanding others. Understanding others was difficult even for King Yao and King Yu, who lamented over this matter. So, how can a person be easily satisfied in just knowing others?

There are four types of desires in the human mind. Those who neglect propriety and are self-indulgent are called "Mean." Those who neglect righteousness and seek personal comfort are called "Weak." Those who neglect wisdom and try to deceive others are called "Superficial." Those who neglect benevolence and are overly greedy are called "Avaricious."

Longevity and Life Preservation in Eastern Medicine,
"A Discourse on the Four Principles"

Taeyangins ... can be overly self-indulgent. *Soeumins*... can be overly idle. *Soyangins* ... can be overly partial. *Tae-eumins*... can be overly greedy.

Longevity and Life Preservation in Eastern Medicine,
"A Discourse on the Establishment and Supplement"

(4) Theory of Self-Rectification by Lee Je-ma

Dr. Lee Je-ma's philosophy is based on the spirit of "self-cultivation and governing others" that came from the reinterpretation of the original Confucianism (based on Four Books and Three Classics), with particular emphasis on self-cultivation. "Knowing others and self-rectification" were presented as a method of self-cultivation. This was derived directly from the "spirit of knowledge and conduct" that developed from "insincere conduct and not clearly understanding others." Among them, self-rectification sought its foundation from "insincere conduct."

Dr. Lee Je-ma stated in "Caution on Insincerity" from the book *Manuscript of Science* that "one should constantly reflect on one's path of sincerity and self-admonition." He added, "the proper pursuit of learning is to reflect on sincerity and not to carry out dishonest acts even if one is suddenly tempted by thoughts of dishonesty. Therefore, the path to learning is nothing more than redemption from the self-indulgent mind." Here, the spirit of "reflection on sincerity and self-admonition" and "constant vigilance and self-reflection" is the proper attitude of learning and the way of self-rectification according to Dr. Lee Je-ma's philosophy.

The background of Dr. Lee Je-ma's philosophy originates from Mencius' principle of "regulating the mind to rectify oneself," such as the "spirit of self-reflection," "spirit of self-rectification," and "redemption from self-indulgent mind." He explained "sincerity of mind" in the Heaven, Earth, Fire and Water sections in the chapter "Caution on Insincerity" as vigilance of preserving the mind. He explained "respect for the body" in the Mountain, Lake, Thunder, and Wind sections of the same chapter. Thus we can see that his philosophical background stemmed from Mencius' spirit of "regulating the mind to rectify oneself." He praised Mencius as the most adept person at self-rectification.

Aside from this, in order to explain Confucius' spirit on self-rectification, Dr. Lee Je-ma clarified the method of self-rectification through "self-denial and returning to propriety," "hiding the evil and praising the good," and "careful observation of dishonesty." Based on this, he expressed his own method of self-rectification through "sincerely grasping the center" of mental desires and the "constant vigilance and self-reflection" of sorrow, anger, joy, and pleasure.

We can see that Dr. Lee Je-ma's spirit of self-rectification praises Mencius's ability to "regulate the mind to rectify oneself" more than that of Confucius. He succeeded and amplified Mencius' method of self-rectification and realized his own new method, which stemmed from the spirit of harmonious regulation of the Golden Mean.

Such a spirit of self-rectification, as can be seen in Dr. Lee Je-ma's philosophy, developed into principles of "regulating the mind to minimize any negative influences in treating diseases" and "regulating the mind to improve one's health." Thus his theory became used, in a practical sense, as a form of self-rectification in medicine and everyday life. In other words, his philosophy of "knowing others to rectify oneself" developed into a practical application, which led to the "theory of constitutionally understanding others to rectify oneself." Medical self-rectification according to constitution led to the establishment of SCM, and self-rectification in everyday life led to the theory of health cultivation according to the Sasang constitutions.

Dr. Lee Je-ma valued self-rectification (which emphasizes the elevation of one's character) and preventative health cultivation in daily life more than medical self-rectification (which focuses on treating diseases according to constitutional imbalances). Self-rectification includes practicing the virtues of simplicity, diligence, vigilance, and the expansion of knowledge in daily life to overcome dishonest acts that arise from the strong inclinations toward overdrinking, sensual pleasure, wealth and power that reside in people's minds.

Therefore, if successfully carrying out the "affinity for virtue and dislike for evil," in regards to the "respect for wisdom and following virtue" and "jealousy of the wise and the able," is the ultimate purpose of Dr. Lee Je-ma's philosophy, then "understanding others and rectifying oneself" is its method of practice. Self-rectification should be applied in medicine and in daily life to harmonize and regulate the mind, body, activity and matter.

> The sudden and reckless movements of sorrow, anger, joy and pleasure in the world, arise from insincere conduct and not clearly understanding others.
>
> *Longevity and Life Preservation in Eastern Medicine,*
> "A Discourse on the Four Principles"

> By rectifying oneself and seeking nothing from others, there will be no dissatisfaction. One will not hold a grudge toward Heaven, nor grumble against others.
>
> *Doctrine of the Mean*, Chapter 3

> Great men are those who are able to put all things in their proper order to achieve maximum harmony simply by rectifying themselves.
>
> *Mencius*, Jin Xin, Part I, Verse 19

> If the people you love do not reciprocate affection, reflect and examine your benevolence. If problems arise when governing others, reflect and examine your wisdom. If the

people who you treat cordially do not return the courtesy, reflect and examine your own feelings of respect. When you do not realize what you desire by your actions, you must reflect and examine yourself in every way. When a person is righteous, the entire kingdom will turn to him with recognition and respect.

Mencius, Li Lau, Part I, Verse 4

Only after one cultivates oneself like Mencius can one dislike evil without fault.

Manuscript of Science, "Self cultivation"

From childhood to old age, I had many dishonest thoughts. When I carried out those dishonest acts, they led to failure every time, and I became severely distressed. Inevitably, I reflected on the path of sincerity and practiced self-vigilance.

Manuscript of Science, "Caution on Insincerity"

When there is a rise of dishonest thoughts and the acts are carried out, it is indeed falsehood. When there is a rise of dishonest thoughts yet the acts are not carried out, and instead the sincerity of one's conscience is questioned, it is true learning. There is no other way to learn. One just needs to redeem oneself from the self-indulgent mind.

Manuscript of Science, "Caution on Insincerity"

Selfish desires generally reside within the human mind and inevitably they will become attached to wine, women, money and power. This leads one to carry out deceitful acts. Overcoming the strongest desire will diminish the other trivial ones. This is called suppressing selfish desire and returning to righteous behavior.

Manuscript of Science, "Caution on Insincerity"

Confucius said, "King Shun was indeed wise! He loved

to question others, and to learn from their words, which may appear common. He concealed what was bad, and displayed what was good so that people only followed the virtuous deeds. He thoroughly grasped the two extremes of good and evil, determined the most appropriate method, and employed it to govern the people. It was by maintaining the path of the Golden Mean that he became a sage!"

Doctrine of the Mean, Chapter 6

By knowing a person's deceitfulness, his evil can be hidden. By knowing a person's talents, his virtue can be praised. Cunning deceitfulness is difficult to know but talent is readily apparent. By knowing what is difficult, what is easy becomes even easier to know. Thus, being able to know and forgive the deceitful acts of others is more important.

Manuscript of Science, "Caution on Insincerity"

Therefore, investigating matters and extending knowledge involves observing truth or falsehood. The same can be said for having sincerity of thought and rectifying one's mind, and for cultivating the person and regulating the family, and having order in the state and peace throughout the land.

Resenting Heaven and people must have arisen from an inability to see the falsehoods... Alas! The words of Confucius are truly great and right.

Manuscript of Science, "Caution on Insincerity"

One must preserve his or her mental clarity in order to stay vigilant over one's deceitful acts on other people. One should behave properly in order to maintain vigilance over the deceitful acts of others.

Manuscript of Science, "Caution on Insincerity"

If the body indulges in whatever it pleases and the mind is unsettled, it is because one is engaged in a life of debauchery, indolence and greed. This is not a proper way to truly grasp the middle path by following the Golden Mean.

Manuscript of Science, "Caution on Insincerity" "Wind Trigram Section"

Simplicity, diligence, vigilance, and the expansion of knowledge allow one to live a natural life span. When a man respects a woman, sensual pleasures can be enjoyed in an appropriate manner. When a man loves his friends, he will maintain his virtue even when he is out drinking with them. When a man respects a sage, he can utilize power appropriately. When a man cares for the poor, he will do great service with his wealth.

Longevity and Life Preservation in Eastern Medicine, "A Discourse on the General Health Maintenance"

Jealousy of the wise and the able is the most prevalent disease in the world. Respect for the wise and affinity for virtue is the greatest medicine in the world.

Longevity and Life Preservation in Eastern Medicine, "A Discourse on the General Health Maintenance"

(5) Lee Je-ma's Philosophical View of Health

Based on the practical spirit of Confucianism, Dr. Lee Je-ma regarded the human beings to be active and self-regulating beings who emphasize the rebuking of their minds and bodies. So, he viewed health as a state of mind in which there are no desires. This can be achieved by overcoming the desires of the mind.

The mind without desires does not mean that there is a complete absence of desires as is the case in the state of nothingness or enlightenment that was achieved by Lao Tzu or Buddha. Instead, it implies a state of mind in which one constantly worries whether or not the world is governed with compassion, which leaves no room for selfish desires. This is the extremely unselfish state of mind that is acquired through overcoming selfish desires, like the benevolent and altruistic spirit of "learning without losing your thirst for knowledge and teaching without being tired" as practiced by King Yao, King

Shun, Confucius, and Mencius. This is what Dr. Lee Je-ma refers to as a state of health.

The ears, eyes, mouth, and nose or Lungs, Spleen, Liver, and Kidneys of Yao and Shun are the same as those of commoners. However, since Yao and Shun's attributes are not covered by selfish desires, the functions of hearing, seeing, smelling, and tasting of the ears, eyes, nose, and mouth, as well as the learning, inquiring, thinking, and differentiating of the Lungs, Spleen, Liver, and Kidneys manifest properly. These attributes do not function properly in commoners, however, since their ears, eyes, mouth, nose, and Lungs, Spleen, Liver, and Kidneys are covered by selfish desires. Therefore Dr. Lee Je-ma advised vigilance over selfish desires.

States of mental desire directly affect physiological functions, thereby demonstrating the relationship between mind and body. Dr. Lee Je-ma stated that a person's selfishness and desires arise from the "flexion, extension, movement and stillness" of the body and the "will, intention, *hon* (ethereal soul) and *baek* (corporeal soul)" of the mind. The difference between a great person and an inferior person results from differences in their selfish desires.

The goal of a great person is to create order in the state and peace throughout the land, while the inferior person concentrates on creating personal wealth. Thus, the essence, spirit, *qi,* and blood of the great person are profound and vast, while those of the inferior person are superficial and narrow. Furthermore if a person listens extensively, sees expansively, smells broadly and tastes deeply so as to make the function of ears, eyes, nose, and mouth profound, this will create essence, spirit, *qi* and blood, which may be exhausted in a superficial and narrow-minded person. If the functions of the Lungs, Spleen, Liver and Kidneys are upright and harmonious because of proper learning, inquiring, thinking and differentiating, then there will be sufficient *jin* (the thin and clear body fluid), *go* (pasty substance), *you* (oily substance), and *aek* (thick fluid). However, if the functions of the organs are unbalanced and disharmonious, *jin*, *go*, *you*, and *aek* will be consumed.

As previously mentioned, Dr. Lee Je-ma makes no distinction between the health of the body and the health of the mind. He views the mind and body as a single unit in regards to health, but emphasizes mental attributes.

Additionally, he states that a person should practice simplicity, diligence, vigilance, and the expansion of knowledge in order to achieve longevity. To accomplish this, a person must avoid excessive sensual pleasure, he must not drink immoderately or overeat, and he should refrain from the pursuit of power and the accumulation of wealth. Dr. Lee Je-ma also emphasizes the social aspect of health when he suggests that jealousy of the wise and able can cause disease.

Ultimately, Dr. Lee Je-ma's view of health is based on Confucianism as it emphasizes the health of the mind that is acquired by overcoming selfish desires. At the same time, it expresses the mind-body connection to health in which a healthy state of mind is directly linked to physical and physiological health. He also gives weight to the social aspect of health.

> The mind of a sage is said to exist without desire. However, the absence of desire does not imply the state of nothingness or enlightenment that was achieved by Lao Tzu or Buddha. Rather, it implies that the sage is deeply concerned about the chaos of the world, and so has no time for selfish desires. This, in turn, implies that the sage learns without loosing their thirst for knowledge, and teaches without tiring. Learning without loosing their thirst for knowledge and teaching without being tired indicates that the sage has no desires. If even the slightest selfish desire exists in the mind, it cannot be the same mind as Yao and Shun. If the mind, even for a moment, has no concern for the world, it is not the same mind as Confucius and Mencius.
>
> *Longevity and Life Preservation in Eastern Medicine,*
> "A Discourse on the Four Principles"

> Since Yao and Shun's ears, eyes, nose, and mouth are not masked by selfish desires, their function of hearing, seeing, smelling, and tasting manifest properly, while those of commoners do not function properly since they are masked by selfish desires. Since Yao and Shun's Lungs, Spleen, Liver, and Kidneys are not masked by selfish desires, their

functions of learning, inquiring, thinking, and differentiating manifest properly, while those of commoners do not because they are masked by selfish desires.

Human desires arise from the will, intention, *hon* (ethereal soul), and *baek* (corporeal soul) of the mind, while selfishness arises from the flexion, extension, movement, and stillness of the body. The will, intention, *hon* and *baek* of a great person are focused on bringing order to the state and making peace throughout the land. Thus his essence, spirit, *qi,* and blood are profound and vast. But those of an inferior person are superficial and narrow since his focus is on accumulating family wealth and building a prominent career for himself. The sincere mind and reverent behavior of a great person control his bodily flexion, extension, movement and stillness. So his trunk, head, and limbs are akin to a ruler that is able to draw a circle, triangle, or horizontal lines, as well as, a carpenter's inkline. But the self-indulgent mind and idle behavior of an inferior person control his bodily flexion, extension, movement, and stillness. So his trunk, head, and limbs are unlike the ruler and the carpenter's inkline.

Manuscript of Science, "Self-cultivation"

The ears must listen extensively, the eyes must see expansively, the nose must smell broadly, and the mouth must taste deeply. When the functions of the ears, eyes, nose and mouth are profound and vast, essence, spirit, *qi,* and blood will be created. Otherwise, if they are superficial and narrow, essence, spirit, *qi,* and blood will be exhausted.

The Lungs must excel at learning. The Spleen must excel at inquiring. The Liver must excel at thinking. The Kidneys must excel at differentiating. When the functions of Lungs, Spleen, Liver and Kidneys are upright and harmonious, the *jin* (the thin and clear body fluid), *go* (pasty substance), *you* (oily substance), and *aek* (thick fluid) will be sufficient. If the functions of the organs are unbalanced and disharmonious, *jin*, *go*, *you*, and *aek* will be consumed.

Longevity and Life Preservation in Eastern Medicine,
"A Discourse on the Viscera and Bowels"

Simplicity, diligence, vigilance, and the expansion of knowledge allow one to live one's natural life span. The simple person avoids sensual pleasure. The diligent person avoids overdrinking. The vigilant person avoids the pursuit of power. The wise person avoids accumulating wealth.

Jealousy of the wise and the able is the most prevalent disease in the world. Respect for the wise and affinity for virtue is the greatest medicine in the world.

Longevity and Life Preservation in Eastern Medicine,
"A Discourse on General Health Maintenance"

(6) Lee Je-ma's Viewpoint of the Constitution

Dr. Lee Je-ma stated that he was born approximately 5,000 years after the first historically known medical experience and that he discovered the principle of the four organs of the Sasang constitutions by chance through the writings of ancient doctors. Through this discovery he clarified the congenital attributes of human beings into the four constitutions.

These congenital attributes allow people to be classified into constitutions based on the size of four organs. A person with large Lungs and a small Liver is called *Taeyangin*, while a person with a large Liver and small Lungs is called *Tae-eumin*. A person with a large Spleen and small Kidneys is called *Soyangin* while a person with large Kidneys and a small Spleen is called *Soeumin*. Dr. Lee Je-ma states that the sizes of the organs are reflected by the nature and emotions of the Sasang constitutions. He also divides human nature or disposition into benevolence, righteousness, propriety, and wisdom, and mental desires or inclinations into rudeness, superficiality, greed and indolence. Based on these distinctions, he explains the differences between a sage and a commoner. In addition, he differentiates the mental desires of the Sasang constitutions by labeling a person who throws away propriety and does whatever he pleases, "Mean" (*Taeyangin*); a person who throws away righteousness and pursues his own comfort, "Weak" (*Soeumin*); a person who throws away wisdom and subtly tries to deceive others, "Superficial" (*Soyangin*); and a person who throws away benevolence and is extremely greedy, "Avaricious" (*Tae-eumin*).

The theory of the different sized organs encompasses not only the idea that the organs are of varying physical sizes and that their functions have different excesses and deficiencies, it also maintains that there is a variation in the magnitude of dispersing *qi*, gathering *qi*, accumulating *qi*, and releasing *qi* in the organs. In particular, these variations explain the functions of the four organs in relation to the movements of *qi* (straight rising, obliquely ascending, obliquely descending and straight dropping), according to the ascending and descending movements of the four emotions (sorrow, anger, joy, and pleasure).

SCM places more emphasis on the function of the smaller organs when discussing the attributes of the four organs. For instance, the large Kidneys and small Spleen of *Soeumins* represent the organ's characteristics that will manifest as excessive releasing *qi* and deficient accumulating *qi*. The upper mid-back region and the Stomach, which belong to the smaller Spleen, become the foundation (interior), while the Bladder and the Large Intestine of the larger Kidneys are the manifestation (exterior). The factor essential to preserving the life of *Soeumins* is the maintenance of the warm *yang qi*. The other constitutions can be explained in the same manner. Clear *yin qi* is the essential component for the preservation of *Soyangins*, for *Tae-eumins* it is dispersing *qi* and for *Taeyangins* it is gathering *qi*.

Dr. Lee Je-ma also explained the nature and emotions of the Sasang constitutions. The peculiarities of the natures of each constitution are as follows: *Taeyangins* tend to move forward and not backwards. *Soyangins* tend to be active but do not pause to think. *Tae-eumins* tend to be still and not active. *Soeumins* tend to remain in one place and do not go out.

The attributes of the emotions of each constitution are that *Taeyangins* tend to be masculine and not feminine, while *Soeumins* tend to be feminine and not masculine. *Soyangins* strive toward external achievements and do not maintain their domestic affairs, while *Tae-eumins* strive toward maintaining their domestic affairs but not toward external achievements.

The nature of the Sasang constitutions forms the basis for their "constant state of mind" as well as for their "talents and skills." The emotions of the Sasang constitutions give rise to passions such as self-indulgence, partiality, idleness, and selfish desire. These then cause the mental desires of rudeness, superficiality, greed, and indolence, while bringing about the psychological states of explosive anger, stirring of sorrow, unrestrained pleasure, and, unstable joy.

Because these natures and emotions are congenital, people should remain vigilant and introspective to overcome these attributes and establish harmony. If the nature and emotions are even slightly out of balance they will manifest as mental desires. Thus, variances in sorrow, anger, joy and pleasure were cautioned according to individual constitutions. For example, *Taeyangins* are told to guard against explosive anger and deep sorrow, *Soyangins* against sudden sorrow and deep anger, *Tae-eumins* against fluctuating pleasure and deep joy, and *Soeumins* against fluctuating joy and deep pleasure.

During his explanations of the principles of the organs, mental desires, nature and emotions, Dr. Lee Je-ma makes no claim of the superiority of one constitution over any of the others. His only comparison is between the sage and the commoner. The strengths and weaknesses of the four organs exist in the same proportions whether a person is sage-like or common because of Heaven's principles of nature. The organ relationships are inherent and cannot be changed. It is the clarity of mind and magnitude of mental desires that differentiate the sage from the commoner. This difference is not inherent but is determined through the practice of self-cultivation in daily life.

According to Dr. Lee Je-ma's view of the constitutions, even a sage can be classified according to his constitutional type. In addition, it is possible for a commoner to become a sage. The attributes of the organs' principles and the nature and emotions of each constitution were explained based on the principles of self-regulation and self-restraint and on the practical spirit of Confucianism.

> Human beings are born with four differing principles of organs. A person with large Lungs and a small Liver is called *Taeyangin*. A person with a large Liver and small Lungs is called *Tae-eumin*. A person with a large Spleen and

small Kidneys is called *Soyangin*. And a person with large Kidneys and a small Spleen is called *Soeumin*.

In *Taeyangins*, the nature of sorrow is distantly dispersed and the emotion of anger is urgent. When sorrow is distantly dispersed, the *qi* flows into the Lungs and they become even more exuberant. When anger is urgent, the *qi* violently stimulates the Liver and it becomes further depleted. Thus the *Taeyangins*' organ formation is large Lungs and a small Liver. In *Soyangins*, the nature of anger is widely encompassed and the emotion of sorrow is urgent. When anger is widely encompassed, the *qi* flows into the Spleen and it becomes even more exuberant. When sorrow is urgent, the *qi* violently stimulates the Kidneys, and it becomes further depleted. Thus the *Soyangins*' organ formation is a large Spleen and small Kidneys. In *Tae-eumins*, the nature of joy extends broadly and the emotion of pleasure is urgent. When joy extends broadly, the *qi* flows into the Liver and it becomes even more exuberant. When pleasure is urgent, the *qi* violently stimulates the Lungs and they become further depleted. Thus the *Tae-eumins*' organ formation is a large Liver and small Lungs. In *Soeumins*, the nature of pleasure is deep and the emotion of joy is urgent. When pleasure is deep, the *qi* flows into the Kidneys and they become even more exuberant. When joy is urgent, the *qi* violently stimulates the Spleen and it becomes further depleted. Thus the *Soeumins*' organ formation is large Kidneys and a small Spleen.

There are four human desires. Those who throw away propriety and do whatever they please are called "Mean." Those who throw away righteousness and pursue their own comfort are called "Weak." Those who throw away wisdom and subtly try to deceive others are called "Superficial." And those who throw away benevolence and are extremely greedy are called "Avaricious."

Longevity and Life Preservation in Eastern Medicine,
"A Discourse on the Four Principles"

It is the nature of *Taeyangins* to always move forward but not backwards. It is the nature of *Soyangins* to be active but not to finish what they have begun. It is the nature of *Tae-eumins* to be still and not active. And it is the nature of *Soeumins* to remain in one place and not go out.

The emotional character of *Taeyangins* tends to be masculine and not feminine. The emotional character of *Soeumins* tends to be feminine but not masculine. The emotional character of *Soyangins* strives towards external achievements but not toward maintaining their domestic affairs. The emotional character of *Tae-eumins* strives toward maintaining their domestic affairs but not toward external achievements.

Though *Taeyangins* tend to be masculine, it is advisable for them to be feminine to some extent. If they become totally masculine, they will become excessively self-indulgent. Though *Soeumins* tend to be feminine, it is advisable for them to be masculine to some extent. If they become totally feminine, they will become excessively idle. Though *Soyangins* strive toward external achievements, it is advisable for them to maintain their domestic affairs to some extent. If they only strive toward external achievements, they will become overly partial towards internal achievements. Though *Tae-eumins* strive toward maintaining their domestic affairs, it is advisable for them to strive toward external achievements to some extent. If they only strive toward maintaining their domestic affairs, they will become excessively greedy.

Longevity and Life Preservation in Eastern Medicine,
"A Discourse on the Establishment and Supplement"

Although four different categories of organ formations exist, the one thing common to all four categories is the transformation of the principles of nature. This is why the sage and the commoner are identical. Although four different classes of the mind exist, there are 10,000 different levels in each class due to the magnitude of selfish desires. This is why the sage and the commoner are different in 10,000 ways.

The strengths and weaknesses of the four organs occur because of the changes of *yin* and *yang*. Thus, there is no need to mention how people's disposition is inherently determined. Yet variations exist in the strengths and weaknesses of the organs such that people's inherent dispositions become incomplete. The destiny of such people is dependent upon how well they cultivate themselves in their daily lives. This must be cautioned.

Taeyangins have a tendency toward explosive anger and deep sorrow, to which they must remain vigilant. *Soyangins* have a tendency toward sudden sorrow and deep anger, to which they must remain vigilant. *Tae-eumins* have a tendency towards fluctuating pleasure and deep joy, to which they must remain vigilant. *Soeumins* have a tendency toward fluctuating joy and deep pleasure, to which they must remain vigilant.

Taeyangins and *Soyangins* should remain vigilant toward excessive sorrow and anger. Forcing joy and pleasure upon themselves would be done in vain because their joy and pleasure will not be genuine. This would also create an even greater imbalance of sorrow and anger. *Tae-eumins* and *Soeumins* should remain vigilant toward excessive joy and pleasure. Forcing sorrow and anger upon themselves would be done in vain because their sorrow and anger will not be genuine. This would also create an even greater imbalance of joy and pleasure.

If sorrow, anger, joy and pleasure are not stirred within, then one is in a state of equilibrium. If they manifest in an appropriate manner then one is in a state of harmony. A person who does not express sorrow, anger, joy, and pleasure, yet who is constantly vigilant of his emotions, will he not gradually become similar to a person who is in a state of equilibrium? And a person who expresses sorrow, anger, joy, and pleasure yet reflects upon them, is he not similar to a person who is in a state of harmony?

Longevity and Life Preservation in Eastern Medicine,

"A Discourse on the Four Principles"

In large Lungs, there is excessive dispersing *qi*, while in a small Liver, there is deficient gathering *qi*. In a large Liver, there is excessive gathering *qi*, while in small Lungs, there is insufficient dispersing *qi*. In a large Spleen, there is excessive accumulating *qi*, while in small Kidneys, there is insufficient releasing *qi*. In large Kidneys, there is excessive releasing *qi*, while in a small Spleen, there is insufficient accumulating *qi*.

In *Taeyangins*, the essential component to sustaining life is the gathering *qi*. Thus the waist and Small Intestine are the foundation, while the head/neck and Esophagus are the manifestations. In *Tae-eumins*, the essential component to sustaining life is the dispersing *qi*. Thus the head/neck and Esophagus are the foundation, while waist and Small Intestine are the manifestations. In *Soyangins*, the essential component to sustaining life is the clear *yin qi*. Thus the Bladder and Large Intestine are the foundation while upper mid-back and Stomach are the manifestations. In *Soeumins*, the essential component to sustaining life is the warm *yang qi*. Thus the upper mid-back and Stomach are the foundations, while Bladder and Large Intestine are manifestations.

Lee Je-ma, *Self-Annotation*

(7) Lee Je-ma's Viewpoint of the Pathology

Dr. Lee Je-ma claims that, in the past, most doctors believed that diseases developed from injury to the Spleen and Stomach from inappropriate foods, or by an invasion of climatic factors such as wind, cold, heat and dampness. He states that these doctors did not know that diseases could arise from an imbalance of emotions such as love, hate, desire, joy, anger, sadness and pleasure. Thus, he presented the characteristics of sorrow, anger, joy, and pleasure according to the constitutions and clarified how an imbalance of emotions could cause disease.

Under the premise of mutual interaction between nature and human beings, traditional Syndrome Medicine holds the view that disease is caused by "excessive pathogenic *qi* and deficient righteous *qi*," depending upon whether the focus is on the pathogenic factor or the Source (*Yuan*) *qi*. Dr. Lee Je-ma, however, on the basis of humanity centered reasoning, viewed the development of diseases as a tilt of innate nature and emotions according to an imbalance of sorrow, anger, joy and pleasure that directly influenced the internal organs, and not as an interplay between Righteous *qi* and pathogenic *qi*.

Dr. Lee Je-ma also stated that the *qi* of sorrow and anger rise upward and if they do so in a reckless manner, the Liver and Kidneys in the Lower Burner will be injured. He said that the *qi* of joy and pleasure descend, but if they do so in a reckless manner, the Lungs and the Spleen in the Upper Burner will be injured. Furthermore, he stated that if *Taeyangins*' sorrow becomes extreme, anger will spring forth. If *Soyangins*' anger becomes extreme, sorrow will stir deeply within. If *Soeumins*' pleasure becomes extreme, joy becomes unstable. If *Tae-eumins*' joy becomes extreme, pleasure becomes unrestrained. Thus, Dr. Lee Je-ma explained how unbalanced emotions could be an important factor in causing a disease in each constitution.

In addition, Dr. Lee Je-ma said that when children become ill, their affectionate mothers should protect them. When young adults become ill, their wise fathers or intelligent older brothers should protect them. When adults become ill, their younger brothers or good friends should support them. When elders become ill, their offspring or grandchildren should support them. If a person living in a mountain is without knowledge, or a person living in a city is without simplicity, or a person living in countryside is without diligence, or an intellectual is without vigilance, these people will have the misfortune of a short life span. Therefore, Dr. Lee Je-ma made the claim that discord in social relationships according to age and time, or disharmony between place and environment can bring about disease.

Furthermore the immoral mind and idle conduct, such as overindulging in luxuries, laziness, partiality, and greed can be life threatening. These will naturally be followed by overdrinking, excessive sensual pleasure, the accumulation of wealth and struggles for power that are like imprisonment. If these four vices become excessive, many evil people will gather in the homes of the offenders and their offspring and wives will become ill. He explained that all diseases result from being jealous of the wise and the able. And the cure for all diseases in this world is to love wisdom and to enjoy doing what is good.

Dr. Lee Je-ma's view of pathology can be summed up in two ways. The first is a pathological view based upon innate nature and emotions, in which diseases develop from an imbalance of innate nature and emotion due to excesses and deficiencies of the four emotions according to individual constitutions. The second is a pathological view according to morals and ethics, in which diseases develop from disharmonious personal and social relationships according to age, job and lifestyle, as well as, imbalances from alcoholic drinks, sensual pleasure, the accumulation of wealth, and struggles for power. The former is a pathological view according to the constitutions, which centers on innate nature and emotion and places an emphasis on the treatment of diseases. The latter is the pathological view according to the general rule of health cultivation in the daily lives of all people. It is based upon the practical ethics of Confucianism.

> Most doctors in the past did not understand that diseases arise from an imbalance of the emotions of the mind such as love, hate, desire, joy, anger, sadness and pleasure. Instead they thought that diseases develop from injury to the Spleen and Stomach due to inappropriate foods, or by an invasion of climatic factors such as wind, cold, heat and dampness. Their theories regarding disease and medicine were primarily focused on methods to treat diseases arising from dietary imbalances caused by a deficiency of the Spleen and Stomach in *Soeumins*...
>
> *Longevity and Life Preservation in Eastern Medicine,*
> "A Discourse on the Origin of Eastern Medicine"

> Before the age of seven or eight, children may develop illnesses due to a stagnation of the four emotions (sorrow, anger, joy and pleasure) stemming from a lack of knowledge. Thus, they need to be cared for by their affectionate mothers. Before the age of 24 or 25, young adults can get sick from a stagnation of the four emotions stemming from a lack of

courage. Thus, they need to be protected by their wise fathers or intelligent older brothers. During adulthood before the age of 38 or 39, support should come from a sensible younger brothers or good friends. During old age before 56 or 57, help should come from their offspring or grand children.

If a person living in the mountains is without knowledge, or a person living in a city is without simplicity, or a person living in countryside is without diligence, or an intellectual is without vigilance, they will have the misfortune of a short life span.

The home of a virtuous person attracts other virtuous people whereas the home of an immoral person attracts other immoral people. A gathering of many virtuous people activates the virtuous energy of their organs while a gathering of many immoral people arouses the immoral energy of their minds. Since many immoral people gather in houses where there is overindulgence in alcoholic drinks and sex, and pursuit of wealth and power, their offspring and wives will become afflicted with diseases.

Overdrinking, sensual pleasure, wealth and power have been cautioned since ancient times and were compared to the constraints of four walls of a jail. These four vices influence not only one's longevity and family fortune, but also the maintenance of a society.

Overindulgence in luxury can shorten one's life span. Indolence can shorten one's life span. Partiality can shorten one's life span. Greed can shorten one's life span. The overindulgent person will surely indulge in sensual pleasure. The idle person will surely immerse himself in drinking. The prejudiced person will surely struggle for power. The greedy person will surely die for the pursuit of money and wealth.

To make a household harmonious, one must love wisdom and follow virtue. A household which is not harmonious has within it the jealousy and hate of the wise and the able people. Generally, if illnesses plague a household, and death often follows, and children become foolish, and the property becomes ruined, it is due to a jealousy and hatred of the wise and the able by the foolish husband and jealous wife.

Longevity and Life Preservation in Eastern Medicine,
"A Discourse on the General Health Maintenance"

If the *qi* of sorrow and anger move in a reckless manner, they will ascend explosively and gather in the upper body. If the *qi* of joy and pleasure move in a reckless manner, they will descend violently and gather in the lower body. When the ascending *qi* moves in a reckless manner to gather in the upper body, the Liver and Kidneys are injured. When the descending *qi* moves in a reckless manner to gather in the lower body, the Spleen, and the Lungs are injured.

If *Taeyangins*' sorrow becomes extreme, anger will spring forth. If *Soyangins*' anger becomes extreme, sorrow will stir deeply within. If *Soeumins*' pleasure becomes extreme, joy becomes unstable. If *Tae-eumins*' joy becomes extreme, pleasure becomes unrestrained. Such a strong stirring of emotions can be compared to cutting one's intestines with a knife so that 10 years will not be enough time to recover one's health. This will determine life and death, longevity and premature death. That is why it must never be forgotten.

Longevity and Life Preservation in Eastern Medicine,
"A Discourse on the Four Principles"

Appendix 3

Fundamental Concepts of Sasang Constitutional Medicine

(1) The Ontology of Sasang Philosophy

Dr. Lee Je-ma named the four Sasang constitutions; *Taeyangin*, *Soyangin*, *Tae-eumin* and *Soeumin* and explained their differences in the chapter, "A Discourse on Four Principles" found in *Longevity and Life Preservation in Eastern Medicine.*

In the context of SCM, "Sasang" implies four different patterns of material phenomena that are based on the spirit of simplification that exists within the four substance classifications. This meaning of Sasang is slightly different to the one found in the *I Ching* in which Sasang represents the symbols that express variance of *yin* and *yang*.

In the "Great Treatise" (Great Essays) of the *I Ching* it is said, "Within the principles of the *I Ching* is the *taichi*, the Supreme Ultimate. *Taichi* begets the Two Modes, *yin* and *yang*. The Two Modes generate the Sasang (Four Symbols/ Images). The Sasang generates the Eight Trigrams. The Eight Trigrams determine fortune and misfortune. Fortune and misfortune create the great field of action that will decide success or failure." Thus trigrams, which represent various phenomena, are created after undergoing three stages of transformation from *taichi* to Two Modes to Sasang and finally to the Eight Trigrams. This is the meaning of the Eight Trigrams that is emphasized in the *I Ching*. In SCM, however, the differentiation of the Sasang is explained through the contrasting concepts of "matter" and "principle." The *taichi* and Two Modes correspond to "principle," while Sasang corresponds to "matter." The Sasang is thus seen as the concrete, material phenomenon that does not further differentiate, and is considered to be the basic unit of all things in nature.

We can interpret such an ontological meaning of the Sasang from the perspective of "substance" and "function." Dr. Lee Je-ma states in the chapter "Caution on Insincerity" from his book *Manuscript of Science* that, "The *taichi* is the mind. The Two Modes are the mind and body. Sasang is the activity, mind, body, and matter. The Eight

Trigrams are the beginning and end of activity, the root and branch of matter, the moderation and urgency of the mind, and the congenital and acquired aspects of the body." Thus Dr. Lee Je-ma clarified the ontological meaning of Sasang by comparing it to the above-mentioned differentiation process in the "Great Treatise (Great Essays)" of *I Ching*. This can be understood from the perspective of "substance." In other words, the essence of all things has, as a basic unit of constituent elements, the material phenomena of Sasang, which are activity, mind, body and matter. The Eight Trigrams are merely the dual aspects of *yin* and *yang* of the Sasang.

Meanwhile, in a draft of his SCM book, Dr. Lee Je-ma explains the *taichi*, Two Modes and *Sasang* in the following way, which can be interpreted from the perspective of "function."

> "Heaven created all things in nature, and all things have a material aspect and a principle aspect. The human body corresponds to *matter*, while human nature corresponds to *principle*. When a bodily form exists, so does human nature, and when matter exists, so does its principle. Thus, that which is one and not two is called *taichi*. Human nature has an application. The application of nature is knowledge. The human body also has an application. The application of the body is its conduct. With knowledge comes conduct, with creation comes development. Thus, through the principle of mutual exchange, one acquires the other. This is called the Two Modes. Within knowledge are extension and contraction. Extension implies a decision while contraction implies a perception. Within conduct are progression and regression. Progression implies movement while regression implies stoppage. That which has changes and stillness, as well as, movement and transformation, such as decision and perception, movement and stoppage, extension and contraction, progression and regression, is called Sasang."
>
> *Draft of Sasang Constitutional Medicine*, Chapter 4

Thus, Dr. Lee Je-ma explained the *taichi* as the integrated state in which matter and principle, or *form* and *nature* are one and the same.

The Two Modes are defined as knowledge and conduct, or creation and development. Sasang can be understood as the relationship between movement and stillness, change and transformation that manifest as extension, contraction, progression, and regression, or decision, perception, movement, and stoppage.

Through these associations, the ontological perspective of Sasang philosophy can be interpreted as the relationship between form and function. Accordingly, the meaning of Sasang in SCM can be considered to be the summation of the constituent and transforming elements of all things in nature into a four-substance classification.

Meanwhile, we can look to the following comments from the *Doctrine of the Mean* to explain the basic concepts of Dr. Lee Je-ma's Sasang philosophy, as it stems from the spirit of Confucianism.

> "In this world, it requires the utmost sincerity for a person to fully develop his nature. When a person fully develops his nature, he can do the same for the nature of others. By fully developing the nature of others, he can fully develop the nature of all things."
>
> *Doctrine of the Mean*, Chapter 22

> "A person with sincerity not only completes himself, he also completes other things in nature. Self-completion is benevolence, while completing other things in nature is knowledge. Sincerity is the way of Heaven thus benevolence and knowledge are virtues that belong to one's nature. Sincerity is also the way to unify both the interior (oneself) and the exterior (all things in nature). Therefore, a person should always be sincere."
>
> *Doctrine of the Mean*, Chapter 25

> "If sorrow, anger, joy and pleasure are not stirred within, then one is in a state of equilibrium. If they manifest in an appropriate manner then one is in a state of harmony. This equilibrium is the foundation of all matter and phenomena in nature, while harmony is the Tao that should be pursued by all matter and phenomena in nature. Therefore, when

equilibrium and harmony exist in perfection, order will be established throughout Heaven and Earth (all things and phenomena in nature) and all things will be nourished in a harmonious way."

Doctrine of the Mean, Chapter 1

In other words, the evolution of the constituent elements of Sasang (mind, body, activity, and matter) began with the simplification of the self (interior) and matter (exterior), as described in the statements, "fully developing one's nature and all things" and "completing oneself and all things in nature" from the *Doctrine of the Mean*. Then, "self" was expanded to include "mind and body" and "matter" was expanded to include "activity and matter." And with the spirit of "fully developing" (the internal aspect) and "completion" (the external aspect), the "path that unifies both the interior (oneself) and the exterior (all things in nature)" was completed. According to Dr. Lee Je-ma, completion of this path can lead to complete recognition of all matter and phenomena. In addition, Dr. Lee Je-ma explained that the internal phenomena of *taichi* and the Two Modes is the "principle" while the external phenomena of Sasang is "matter."

In Dr. Lee Je-ma's view, the sorrow, anger, joy and pleasure inherent in human nature are the *taichi*. Equilibrium and harmony are the Two Modes. Meanwhile "establishing order throughout Heaven and Earth and nourishing all things in a harmonious way," is the phenomenon of Sasang. Thus, he suggests that Sasang, in the form of "matter," manifest as the result of *taichi* and the Two Modes, which are the "principle." Therefore, the ontological perspective of Sasang philosophy has its basis in the spirit of Confucianism, which includes the *Doctrine of the Mean.*

In summary, the association between "*taichi*, the Two Modes and Sasang" is interpreted as a "vertical cognitive system" that can be used to interpret the relationship between the "principle" (the interior, causative, principle aspects) and "matter" (the exterior, resultant, actualized aspects) according to the ontological relationship of Sasang philosophy. The four-substance classification of Sasang, on the other hand, is viewed as a "horizontal cognitive system," which can be interpreted from the perspective of "substance" (constituent element) and "application" (transforming element). Therefore, it is only by understanding the structural relationship of Sasang while simultaneously applying the horizontal and vertical cognitive systems, that the true meaning of Sasang can be retained. In other words, the spirit of "principle and matter" exists simultaneously within the inner aspect of the four-element structure ontology, while the philosophical perspective of "principle and matter" emerges in the medical perspective as "Interior *qi*, Exterior Form." Thus we can understand this inseparable interdependence of structure (form) and function (*qi*).

The cognitive system of TCM is based on the workings of the Five Elements and the simplification of all things into a five-substance classification. It therefore explains the Five Element Organ Theory, the Five Organ Pathology, the Five Phase Circuit, the Six Energies Theory, and the Five Types of People Theory, etc. This theory emphasizes the Five Element classifications and does not give weight to the spirit of "principle and matter." In contrast, the cognitive system of SCM classifies all things into four substances and, simultaneously, explores the cognitive system of form or shape based on the spirit of "principle and substance." The importation of such a new cognitive system enabled the systematization of a complete constitutional concept that included bodily shape and the principle of the internal organs of each Sasang constitution. It also served as the background by which SCM developed into a mind-body balancing medicine.

(2) The Theory of Human Nature and the Nature-Order of Sasang Philosophy

Confucianism teaches that heaven bestows upon human beings their nature. The first chapter of the *Doctrine of the Mean* states, "That which is bestowed by heaven to human beings is called *nature*; acting in accordance with this nature is called Tao; and the cultivation of Tao is called teaching." Thus, in order to fulfill the *nature* that is bestowed by heaven, one must "fully develop the *nature* of oneself and others," as well as, "fully develop the *nature* of all things." Neo-Confucianist philosopher Zhu Xi reinterpreted the phrase, "That which is bestowed by heaven to human beings is called nature" into "nature is the principle," thus developing the foundation of Neo-Confucianism from the perspective of "The Theory of the

Organizing Principle." However, while Confucianism spoke only of one's nature, Dr. Lee Je-ma, in the chapter "A Discourse on Nature and Order" from *Longevity and Life Preservation in Eastern Medicine*, explains that when human beings are born they receive not only their *nature* but also their *order* (destiny). He, thereby, elected to take a different position than the one already established. As such, it is more appropriate to view the "theory of human nature" of the Sasang philosophy as a "theory of humanity according to *nature* and *order*."

In "A Discourse on Nature and Order," Dr. Lee Je-ma labeled human nature "common wisdom" and said that all virtuous qualities such as benevolence, righteousness, propriety, wisdom, loyalty, filial piety, friendship and fraternal love correspond to common wisdom, which is also the source of virtue. He considered *order* to be means of livelihood and the origin of the Tao. Professions such as scholar, farmer, craftsman, merchant, and the places where one's life and profession take place such as fields, houses, states, and countries correspond to these means of livelihood. According to this, all human beings are born with good *nature* (common wisdom) and everyone has the talent and means (of livelihood) to manage their own lives. Thus, by cultivating common wisdom and the means of livelihood, Tao and virtue can be completely realized.

Dr. Lee Je-ma explained the relationship between the universe and human beings as a four-element structure consisting of "heaven, human beings, nature and order." He placed human beings at the center and explained that externally occurring phenomena are the "environmental frame" and "human activities," and that internally occurring phenomena are *nature* (common wisdom), and *order* (means of livelihood). Here, the cosmological account of Sasang philosophy is a human-centered theory that interprets universal phenomena with human being's self-regulated will and conduct as the center. This is not the cosmological view of "mutually corresponding heaven and human" relations, in which the human phenomena is a part of the operating principle of the universe or nature, as is seen in Taoism or in the philosophy of the Inner Classic (Nei Jing). Moreover, in the four-element structure (heaven, human beings, nature and order), heaven and human beings are seen as attributes of "matter," while *nature* and *order* are seen as attributes of "principle." Thus we see that Dr. Lee evolves into the state of being of a benevolent sage. Dr. Lee Je-ma thus showed how anyone, regardless of his or her position, could become highly evolved through self-cultivation. Taking personal responsibility and exercising self-control establish the activities of knowledge and conduct that eliminate selfish caring of the mind and body. It is the goal of Dr. Lee Je-ma's theory on human nature, that one may realize the perfection of one's *nature* and *order* through self-regulated knowledge and conduct.

(3) Constitutional Knowledge and Conduct and Treatment Principle of SCM

In "A Discourse on the Four Principles," Dr. Lee Je-ma explained human beings through the differentiation of the Heart, which is the human mind, and the Lungs, Spleen, Liver, and Kidneys, which are the organs of the body. His explanation is based on the perspective of "when matter exists, so does the principle to govern it," which is the relationship between *taichi* and Sasang. He then established the principle that human beings are born with varying sizes of internal organs, and differing degrees of human desire. With this, he explained the differences inherent to the four constitutions.

Dr. Lee Je-ma further explained that the principle of *nature* and the emotions of sorrow, anger, joy, and pleasure reflect the size of the internal organs and the manifestation of their physical shape. All causes of postnatal pathology are also explained through the principle of the ascending and descending of sorrow, anger, joy, and pleasure, thereby explaining the constitutional pathologies. He said, "The sudden or extreme fluctuations of sorrow, anger, joy and pleasure in the world arise from insincere conduct and from not clearly knowing others." So, he considered that the discord between the four emotions must arise from the incompleteness of knowledge and conduct, and stressed that the most effective method to prevent the sudden or extreme fluctuations of the four emotions is through the constitutional knowledge and conduct of the Sasang constitutions.

If sudden or extreme fluctuations of the four emotions are not regulated, sorrow and anger will generate each other and joy and pleasure will complement each other. Thus in *Taeyangins*, anger will violently explode and in *Soyangins* sorrow will stir deeply within. In

Tae-eumins there will be unrestrained pleasure and in *Soeumins* there will be unstable joy. He stated that if any of these phenomena appear even once, it would take ten years for the person to recover from it. This is important when considering the life or death and longevity or shortened life span of a person. Thus, he warned against an imbalance of emotions. He recommended that *Taeyangins* be vigilant over explosive anger and deep sorrow, *Soyangins* over sudden sorrow and deep anger, *Tae-eumins* over fluctuating pleasure and deep joy, and *Soeumins* over fluctuating joy and deep pleasure.

In "A Discourse on the Establishment and Supplement," Dr. Lee Je-ma explained the temperament of the Sasang constitutions to be "moving forward," "being active," "being still," and "remaining in one place." The emotions meanwhile were described as "masculine," "feminine," "having an external orientation (outside achievements)" and "having an internal orientation (domestic affair)." The psychological characteristics of the Sasang constitutions were compared to "external inclination," "internal inclination," "excess," and "deficiency" as described in the book, *Doctrine of the Mean*. *Taeyangins* are inclined toward excess, while *Soeumins* are inclined toward deficiency, *Soyangins* are inclined toward the exterior, while *Tae-eumins* are inclined toward the interior. Thus Dr. Lee Je-ma advised *Taeyangins* to take one-step back, *Soeumins* to take one-step forward, *Soyangins* to observe their inner world, and *Tae-eumins* to observe their outer world. He further advised that the Golden Mean should be maintained in the magnitude of the mind's desires from the perspective of external inclination, internal inclination, excess and deficiency.

Dr. Lee Je-ma described the abilities of the Sasang constitutions in human activities as follows: *Taeyangins* are capable in social acquaintances but not in clanships. *Soyangins* are capable in appointed roles but not in living quarters. *Tae-eumins* are capable in living quarters but not in appointed roles. *Soeumins* are capable in clanships but not in social acquaintances. In order to overcome these tendencies, *Taeyangins* need to eliminate idleness and be diligent in their lives. *Soyangins* need to eliminate extravagance and maintain simplicity in their lives. *Soeumins* need to eliminate their partiality and urgency and must maintain vigilance in their lives. *Tae-eumins* need to throw away their greed and must gain knowledge and information through listening and observing others in their lives. Thus he emphasized the importance of maintaining a balanced external (social) and domestic (personal) life by "the rectification of oneself and the completion of things" in the lives of the Sasang constitutions. When their vices are not overcome, they will fall into lives of over drinking, sensual pleasure, the accumulation of material wealth and struggles for power, which will eventually ruin their lives, damage their health and shorten their life spans.

The above-mentioned are methods to overcome the constitutional weaknesses of the Sasang constitutions. The first is the Golden Mean method of regulating sorrow, anger, joy, and pleasure to overcome the uneven distribution of energy in the body according to the size of the Lungs, Spleen, Liver, and Kidneys. The second is the method to adjust the magnitude of the mental desires by tempering the mental tendencies of external inclination, internal inclination, excess and deficiency in the direction of the Golden Mean. The third is the method to balance external (social) and domestic (personal) obligations by "the rectification of oneself and the completion of things" through the Golden Mean in terms of drinking, sensual pleasure, material wealth and power. This is performed by the Sasang constitutions in order to overcome the inabilities of human activities.

This is Dr. Lee Je-ma's method for maintaining health and his treatment principle of the *Sasang* constitutions that apply the Golden Mean to the body and mind and in social interactions. He then discussed a method for regulating the knowledge and conduct of the Sasang constitutions that epitomizes the Golden Mean for those three areas. In other words, Dr. Lee Je-ma showed that in order for the Sasang constitutions to have the peerless knowledge and conduct of a virtuous person, they must be vigilant of their idle minds and the idle conduct contained within their jaws, chests, navels, and abdomen, as well as, in their heads, shoulders, waists, and hips.

Specifically, Dr. Lee Je-ma warned *Tae-eumins* to be vigilant of arrogance (knowledge) and extravagance (conduct), *Soeumins* of pretentiousness (knowledge) and deprivation (conduct), *Soyangins* of boastfulness (knowledge) and indolence (conduct), and *Taeyangins* of cruelty (knowledge) and pilfering (conduct). He regarded the perfection of knowledge and conduct of the Sasang constitutions to be the most ideal method of overcoming their constitutional weaknesses. When the knowledge of the jaw, chest, navel, and abdomen is correct, the function of the ears, eyes, nose, and mouth becomes profound and vast. Thus essence, spirit, *qi*, and blood are produced and the affinity for virtue becomes greater. When the conduct of the head, shoulders, waist and hips is correct, the function of Lungs, Spleen, Liver and Kidneys becomes upright and centered. Thus *jin* (thin and clear fluids), *go* (pasty substance), *you* (oily substance), and *aek* (thick fluids) become sufficient and the dislike of vices becomes greater.

Therefore, the regulation of knowledge and conduct of the Sasang constitutions is not only a method for maintaining physical health, it also involves the moral principles of "affinity for virtue" and "dislike for vice." As Dr. Lee Je-ma stated, "Being jealous of the wise and the able is the most prevalent disease in the world. And respecting the wise and following virtue is the greatest medicine in the world." The Sasang philosophy can be said to be a medicine that "treats the disease by cultivating the mind" through the regulation of the knowledge and conduct of the Sasang constitutions.

Appendix 4

Constitutional Disease Syndromes and Herbal Formulas

The following classifications contain the complete constitutional disease syndromes of Sasang Constitutional Medicine as they were described in Appendix 1. Each syndrome is matched with a corresponding herbal formula and its ingredients. The formulas that are mentioned are the most frequently used in clinical practice. Some are identical to the traditional formulas of Syndrome Medicine, while others are modifications of traditional formulas. There are also several new formulas that were created by Dr. Lee Je-ma, which he based upon the specific needs of the individual constitutions. The names of all of the formulas are given in English, with their Korean and Chinese versions in parenthesis. Unless otherwise noted, the dosages of the herbs are in grams.

Soeumin Formulas

I. Exterior Diseases

A. Manic Syndrome

1) Initial Stage

- Ligusticum, Angelica, Cyperus and Perilla Powder (*Koong-kwi-hyang-so San/ Xiong-gui-xiang-su San*):

  cyperus (*xiang-fu*) 8, perilla (*zi-su-ye*) 4, ligusticum (*chuan-xiong*) 4, Chinese angelica (*dang-gui*) 4, atractylodes (*cang-zhu*) 4, tangerine peel (*chen-pi*) 4, baked licorice (*zi-gan-cao*) 4, allium (*cong-bai*) 5 stems, fresh ginger (*sheng-jiang*) 3 slices, dates (*da-zao*) 2 pieces

- Ligusticum and Cinnamon Decoction (*Chun-koong-kae-ji Tang/ Chuan-xiong-gui-zhi Tang*):

  cinnamon twig (*gui-zhi*) 12, white peony (*bai-shao*) 8, ligusticum (*chuan-xiong*) 4, atractylodes (*cang-zhu*) 4, tangerine peel (*chen-pi*) 4, baked licorice (*zhi-gan-cao*) 4, fresh ginger (*sheng-jiang*) 3 slices, dates (*da-zao*) 2 pieces

2) Terminal Stage

- Eight Noble Ingredient Decoction (*Pal-mul-keun-ja Tang/ Ba-wu-jun-zi Tang*):

  ginseng (*ren-shen*) 8, astragalus (*huang-qi*) 4, atractylodes (*bai-zhu*) 4, white peony (*bai-shao*) 4, Chinese angelica (*dang-gui*) 4, ligusticum (*chuan-xiong*) 4, tangerine peel (*chen-pi*) 4, baked licorice (*zi-gan cao*) 4, fresh ginger (*sheng-jiang*) 3 slices, dates (*da-zao*) 2 pieces

- All-Inclusive Great Tonifying Decoction (*Ship-chun-dae-bo Tang/ Shi- quan-da-bu Tang*):

  ginseng (*ren-shen*) 4, atractylodes (*bai-zhu*) 4, white peony (*bai-shao*) 4, baked licorice (*zi gan-cao*) 4, astragalus (*huang-qi*) 4, cinnamon bark (*rou-gui*) 4, Chinese angelica (*dang-gui*) 4, ligusticum (*chuan-xiong*) 4, poria (*fu-ling*) 4, cooked rehmannia (*shu-di-huang*) 4, fresh ginger (*sheng-jiang*) 3 slices, dates (*da-zao*) 2 pieces

- Eight Noble Ingredient Decoction with Ginseng (*Dok-sam-pal-mul Tang/ Du-shen-bawu Tang*):

  ginseng (*ren-shen*) 40, astragalus (*huang-qi*) 4, atractylodes (*bai-zhu*) 4, white peony (*bai-shao*) 4, Chinese angelica (*dang-gui*) 4, ligusticum (*chuan-xiong*) 4, tangerine peel (*chen-pi*) 4, baked licorice (*zi-gan-cao*) 4, fresh ginger (*sheng-jiang*) 3 slices, dates (*da-zao*) 2 pieces

B. Collapse of *Yang* Syndrome

1) Initial Stage

- Astragalus and Cinnamon Decoction (*Hwang-ki-kae-ji Tang/ Huang-qi-gui-zhi Tang*):

  cinnamon (*gui-zhi*) 12, white peony (*bai-shao*) 8, astragalus (*huang-qi*) 8, white fleeceflower (*bai-he-shou-wu*) 4, Chinese angelica (*dang-gui*) 4, baked licorice (*zhi-gan-cao*) 4, fresh ginger (*sheng-jiang*) 3 slices, dates (*da-zao*) 2 pieces

- Tonify Middle and Augment the *qi* Decoction (*Bo-joong-yik-ki Tang/ Bu-zhong-yi-qi Tang*):

  ginseng (*ren-shen*) 12, astragalus (*huang-qi*) 12, baked licorice (*zi-gan-cao*) 4, atractylodes (*bai-zhu*) 4, Chinese angelica (*dang-gui*) 4, tangerine peel (*chen-pi*) 4, agastache (*huo-xiang*) 1.2 or 2, perilla (*zi-su-ye*) 1.2 or 2, fresh ginger (*sheng-jiang*) 3 slices, dates (*da-zao*) 2 pieces

- Raise the *yang* and Augment the *qi* Decoction (*Seung-yang-yik-yi Tang/ Sheng-yang-yi-qi Tang*):

  ginseng (*ren-shen*) 8, cinnamon (*gui-zhi*) 8, astragalus (*huang-qi*) 8, white peony (*bai-shao*) 8, white fleeceflower (*bai-he-shou-wu*) 4, cinnamon bark (*rou-gui*) 4, Chinese angelica (*dang-gui*) 4, baked licorice (*zhi-gan-cao*) 4, fresh ginger (*sheng-jiang*) 3 slices, dates (*da-zao*) 2 pieces

2) Terminal Stage

- Astragalus, Cinnamon, and Aconite Decoction (*Hwang-ki-kae-ji-bu-ja Tang/ Huang qi-gui-zhi-fu-zi Tang*):

  cinnamon (*gui-zhi*) 12, astragalus (*huang-qi*) 12, white peony (*bai-shao*) 8, Chinese angelica (*dang-gui*) 4, baked licorice (*zhi-gan-cao*) 4, prepared aconite (*fu-zi*) 4 or 8, fresh ginger (*sheng-jiang*) 3 slices, dates (*da-zao*) 2 pieces

- Ginseng, Cinnamon, and Aconite Decoction (*In-sam-kae-ji-bu-ja Tang/ Ren-shen-gui-zhi-fu-zi Tang*):

  ginseng (ren-shen) 16, cinnamon (*gui-zhi*) 12, white peony (*bai-shao*) 8, astragalus (*huang-qi*) 8, Chinese angelica (*dang-gui*) 4, baked licorice (*zhi-gan-cao*) 4, prepared aconite (*fu-zi*) 2 or 8, fresh ginger (*sheng-jiang*) 3 slices, dates (*da-zao*) 2 pieces

- Raise the *yang* and Augment the *qi* Decoction with Aconite (*Seung-yang-yik-ki-bu-ja Tang/ Sheng-yang-yi-qi-fu-zi Tang*):

  ginseng (*ren-shen*) 8, cinnamon (*gui-zhi*) 8, astragalus (*huang-qi*) 8, white fleeceflower (*bai-he-shou-wu*) 4, cinnamon bark (*rou-gui*) 4, Chinese angelica (*dang-gui*) 4, baked licorice (*zhi-gan-cao*) 4, prepared aconite (*fu-zi*) 2 or 8, fresh ginger (*sheng-jiang*) 3 slices, dates (*da-zao*) 2 pieces

II. Interior Diseases

A. *Tae-eum* Syndrome

- Regulate the Middle Decoction (*Yi-joong-tang/ Li-zhong Tang*):

  ginseng (*ren-shen*) 8, white atractylodes (*bai-zhu*) 8, dried ginger (*gan-jiang*) 8, baked licorice (*zhi-gan-cao*) 4

- Regulate the Middle Decoction with White Fleeceflower and Aconite (*Bak-ha-oh-bu-ja-yi-joong Tang/ Bai-he-wu-fu-zi-li-zhong Tang*):

  white fleeceflower (*bai-he-shou-wu*) 8, white atractylodes (*bai-zhu*) 8, white peony (*bai-shao*) 8, cinnamon twig (*gui-zhi*) 8, dried ginger (*gan-jiang*) 8, tangerine peel (*chen-pi*) 4, baked licorice (*zhi-gan-cao*) 4, prepared aconite (*fu-zi*) 4

- Twelve-Ingredient Decoction to Open the Middle (*Ship-e-mi-kwan-joong Tang/ Shi-er-wei-guan-zhong Tang*):

  white fleeceflower (*bai-he-shou-wu*) 4, red fleeceflower (*chi-he-shou-wu*) 4, galanga (*gao-liang-jiang*) 4, dried ginger (*gan-jiang*) 4, green tangerine peel (*qing-pi*) 4, tangerine peel (*chen-pi*) 4, cyperus (*xiang-fu*) 4, black cardamon (*yi-zhi-ien*) 4, magnolia bark (*hou-po*) 2, immature bitter orange (*zhi-shi*) 2, saussurea (*mu-xiang*) 2, areca peel (*da-fu-pi*) 2, dates (*da-zao*) 2 pieces

- Agastache Powder to Rectify the *qi* (*Kwok-hyang-chung-ki San/ Huo-xiang-zheng-qi San*):

  agastache (*huo-xiang*) 6, perilla (*zi-su-ye*) 4, atractylodes (*cang-zhu*) 2, white atractylodes (*bai-zhu*) 2, pinellia (*ban-xia*) 2, tangerine peel (*chen-pi*) 2, green tangerine peel (*qing-pi*) 2, areca peel (*da-fu-pi*) 2, cinnamon bark (*gui-pi*) 2, dried ginger (*gan-jiang*) 2, black cardamon (*yi-zhi-ren*) 2, baked licorice (*zhi-gan-cao*) 2, fresh ginger (*sheng-jiang*) 3 slices, dates (da-zao) 2 pieces

- Nourish the Stomach Decoction with Cyperus and Cardamon (*Hyang- sa-yang-wi Tang/ Xiang-sha-yang-wei Tang*):

  ginseng (*ren-shen*) 4, white atractylodes (*bai-zhu*) 4, white peony (*bai-shao*) 4, baked licorice (*gan-cao*) 4, pinellia (*ban-xia*) 4, cyperus (*xiang-fu*) 4, tangerine peel (*chen-pi*) 4, dried ginger (*gan-jiang*) 4, hawthorn berry (*shan-zha*) 4, cardamon (*sha-ren*) 4, cluster (*bai-dou-

kou) 4, fresh ginger (*sheng-jiang*) 3 slices, dates (*da-zao*) 2 pieces

- Styrax Pill (*So-hap-hyang-won/ Su-he-xiang-yuan*):

  white atractylodes (*bai-zhu*) 80, saussurea (*mu-xiang*) 80, aquilaria (*chen-xiang*) 80, cloves (*ding-xiang*) 80, santalum (*tan-xiang*) 80, benzoin (*an-xi-xiang*) 80, chebula fruit (*he-zi*) 80, cyperus (*xiang-fu*) 80, long pepper (*bi-ba*) 80, agastache (*huo-xiang*) 80, fennel (*xiao-hui-xiang*) 80, cinnamon bark (*gui-pi*) 80, pteropus (*wu-ling-zhi*) 80, corydalis (*yan-hu-suo*) 40

- Ginseng and Tangerine Peel Decoction (*In-sam-jin-pi Tang/ Ren-shen-chen-pi Tang*):

  ginseng (*ren-shen*) 40, fresh ginger (*sheng-jiang*) 4, cardamon (*sha-ren*) 4, tangerine peel (*chen-pi*) 4, dates (*da-zao*) 2 pieces

B. *Soeum* Syndrome

- Regulate the Middle Decoction with Cinnamon Bark and Aconite (*Kwan-kae-bu-ja-yi-joong Tang/ Guan-gui-fu-zi-li-zhong Tang*):

  ginseng (*ren-shen*) 12, white atractylodes (*bai-zhu*) 8, dried ginger (*gan-jiang*) 8, cinnamon bark (*rou-gui*) 8, white peony (*bai-shao*) 4, tangerine peel (*chen-pi*) 4, baked licorice (*zhi-gan-cao*) 4, aconite (*fu-zi*) 4 or 8

- Regulate the Middle Decoction with Ginseng and Aconite (*Dok-sam-bu-ja-yi-joong Tang/ Du-shen-fu-zi-li-zhong Tang*):

  ginseng (*ren-shen*) 20, white atractylodes (*bai-zhu*) 8, dried ginger (*gan-jiang*) 8, white peony (*bai-shao*) 8, cinnamon bark (*rou-gui*) 8, tangerine peel (*chen-pi*) 4, baked licorice (*zi-gan-cao*) 4, aconite (*fu-zi*) 8, dates (*da-zao*) 2 pieces

- Regulate the Middle Decoction with Evodia and Aconite (*Oh-soo-yu-bu-ja-yi-joong Tang/ Wu-zhu-yu-fu-zi-li-zhong Tang*):

  ginseng (*ren-shen*) 8, white atractylodes (*bai-zhu*) 8, dried ginger (*gan-jiang*) 8, cinnamon bark (*rou-gui*) 8, white peony (*bai-shao*) 4, tangerine peel (*chen-pi*) 4, baked licorice (*zhi-gan-cao*) 4, evodia (*wu-zhu-yu*) 4, fennel (*xiao-hui-xiang*) 4, psoralea (*bu-gu-zhi*) 4, prepared aconite (*fu-zi*) 4 or 8

Soyangin Formulas

I. Exterior Diseases

A. *Soyang* Wind Injury Syndrome

1) *Soyang* Wind Injury Syndrome

- Detoxify Pathogens Decoction with Schizonepata and Sileris (*Hyung- bang-pae-dok San/ Jing-fang-bai-du San*):

  notopterygium (*qiang-huo*) 4, pubescent angelica (*du-huo*) 4, bupleurum (*chai-hu*) 4, peucedanum (*qian-hu*) 4, schizonepeta (*jing-jie*) 4, sileris (*fang-feng*) 4, red poria (*chi-fu-ling*) 4, raw rehmannia (*sheng-di-huang*) 4, lycium bark (*di-gu-pi*) 4, plantain (*che-qian-zi*) 4

2) Knotted Chest Syndrome

- Guide Out the Red Powder with Schizonepeta and Sileris (*Hyung-bang-do-juk San/ Jing-fang-dao-chi San*):

  raw rehmannia (*sheng-di-huang*) 12, plantain (*che-qian-zi*) 8, scrophularia (*xuan-shen*) 6, trichosanthes (*gua-lou-ren*) 6 peucedanum (*qian-hu*) 4, notopterygium (*qiang-hu*)4, pubescent angelica (*du-huo*) 4, schizonepeta (*jing-jie*) 4, sileris (*fang-feng*) 4

- Guide Out the Red and Descend the *qi* Powder (*Do-juk-kang-ki San/ Dao-chi-jiang-qi San*):

  raw rehmannia (*sheng-di*) 12, plantain (*che-qian-zi*) 8, scrophularia (*xuan-shen*) 6, trichosanthes seed (*gua-lou-ren*) 6, peucedanum (*qian-hu*) 4, notopterygium (*qiang-huo*) 4, pubescent angelica (*du-huo*) 4, schizonepata (*jing-jie*) 4, sileris (*fang-feng*) 4, poria (*fu-ling*) 4, alismatis (*ze-xie*) 4

B. Collapse of *Yin* Syndrome

1) Heat of Body/Abdominal Pain + *Yin* Collpase

- Polyporus and Plantain Decoction (*Juh-ryung-cha-jun-ja Tang/ Zhu-ling-che-qian-zi Tang*):

  alismatis (*ze-xie*) 8, poria (*fu-ling*) 8, polyporus (*zhu-ling*) 6, plantain (*che-qian-zi*) 6, anemarrhena (*zhi-mu*) 4, gypsum (*shi-gao*) 4, notopterygium (*qiang-huo*) 4, pubescent angelica (*du-huo*) 4, schizonepeta (*jing-jie*) 4, sileris (*fang-feng*) 4

- Sedate the White Powder with Schizonepeta and Sileris (*Hyung-bang-sa-baek San/ Jing-fang-xie-bai San*):

  raw rehmannia (*sheng-di-huang*) 12, poria (*fu-ling*) 8, alismatis (*ze-xie*) 8, gypsum (*shi-gao*) 4, anemarrhena (*zhi-mu*) 4, notopterygium (*qiang-huo*) 4, pubescent angelica (*du-huo*) 4, schizonepeta (*jing-jie*) 4, sileris (*fang-feng*) 4

2) Coldness of Body/Abdominal Pain + *Yin* Collapse

- Talcum and Sophora Decoction (*Hwal-suk-ko-sam Tang/ Hua-shi-ku-shen Tang*):

  alismatis (*ze-xie*) 8, poria (*fu-ling*) 8, talcum (*hua-shi*) 8, sophora (*ku-shen*) 8, coptis (*huang-lian*) 4, phellodendron (*huang-bai*) 4, notopterygium (*qiang-huo*) 4, pubescent angelica (*du-huo*) 4, schizonepeta (*jing-jie*) 4, sileris (*fang-feng*) 4

- Rehmannia Decoction with Schizonepeta and Sileris (*Hyung Bang Ji Hwang Tang/ Jing Fang Di Huang Tang*):

  cooked rehmannia (*shu-di-huang*) 8, cornus (*shan-zhu-yu*) 8, poria (*fu-ling*) 8, alismatis (*ze-xie*) 8, plantain (*che-qian-zi*) 4, notopterygium (*qiang-huo*) 4, pubescent angelica (*du-huo*) 4, schizonepeta (*jing-jie*) 4, sileris (*fang-feng*) 4

II. Interior Diseases

A. Chest Heat Syndrome

1) Upper Xiao (Wasting and Thirsting Syndrome)

- Cool the Diaphragm and Disperse the Fire Decoction (*yang-gyuk-san-hwa Tang/ Liang-ge-san-huo Tang*):

  raw rehmannia (*sheng-di-huang*) 8, lonicera stem (*ren-tong-teng*) 8, forsythia (*lian-qiao*) 8, gardenia (*zhi-zi*) 4, peppermint (*bo-he*) 4, anemarrhena (*zhi-mu*) 4, gypsum (*shi-gao*) 4, sileris (*fang-feng*) 4, schizonepeta (*jing-jie*) 4

2) Middle Xiao (Wasting and Thirsting Syndrome)

- Lonicera Stem and Lycium Bark Decoction (*In-dong-teung-ji-gol-pi Tang/ Ren-dong-teng-di-gu-pi Tang*):

  lonicera stem (*ren-dong-teng*) 16, cornus (*shan-zhu-yu*) 8, lycium bark (*di-gu-pi*) 8, coptis (*huang-lian*) 4, phellodendron (*huang-bai*) 4, scrophularia (*xuan-shen*) 4, sophora (*ku-shen*) 4, raw rehmannia (*sheng-di-huang*) 4, anemarrhena (*zhi-mu*) 4, gardenia fruit (*zhi-zi*) 4, lycium fruit (*gou-qi-zi*) 4, raspberry (*fu-pen-zi*) 4, schizonepeta (*jing-jie*) 4, sileris (*fang-feng*) 4, lonicera (*jin-yin-hua*) 4

3) Interior Heat Constipation

- White Tiger Decoction with Rehmannia (*Ji-hwang-baek-ho Tang/ Di- huang-bai-hu Tang*):

  gypsum (*shi-gao*) 20 or 40, raw rehmannia (*sheng-di-huang*) 16, anemarrhena (*zhi-mu*) 8, sileris (*fang-feng*) 4, pubescent angelica (*du-huo*) 4

- White Tiger Decoction for Clearing *yang* Toxins (*Yang-dok-bak-ho Tang/ Yang-du-bai-hu Tang*):

  gypsum (*shi-gao*) 20 or 40, raw rehmannia (*sheng-di-huang*) 16, anemarrhena (*zhi-mu*) 8, schizonepeta (*jing-jie*) 4, sileris (*fang-feng*) 4, burdock fruit (*niu-bang-zi*) 4

B. *Yin* Deficiency Tidal Fever Syndrome

1) Lower Xiao (Wasting and Thirsting Syndrome)

- Rehmannia and Sophora Decoction (*Sook-ji-hwang-ko-sam Tang/ Shu- di-huang-ku-shen Tang*):

  cooked rehmannia (*shu-di-huang*)16, cornus (*shan-zhu-yu*) 8, poria (*fu-ling*) 6, alismatis (*ze-xie*) 6, anemarrhena (*zhi-mu*) 4, phellodendron (*huang-bai*) 4, sophora (*ku-shen*) 4

- Six-Ingredient Decoction with Rehmannia (*Yook-mi-ji-hwang Tang/ Liu-wei-di-huang Tang*):

  cooked rehmannia (*shu-di-huang*) 16, dioscorea (*shan-yao*) 8, cornus (*shan-zhu-yu*) 8, alismatis (*ze-xie*) 6, moutan (*mu-dan-pi*) 6, poria (*fu-ling*) 6

2) Stroke, Vomiting, Vomiting of Blood

- Rehmannia Decoction with Pubescent Angelica (*Dok-hwal-ji-hwang Tang/ Du-huo-di-huang Tang*):

  cooked rehmannia (*shu-di-huang*) 16, cornus (*shan-zhu-yu*) 8, poria (*fu-ling*) 6, alismatis (*ze-xie*) 6, moutan (*mu-dan-pi*) 4, sileris (*fang-*

feng) 4, pubescent angelica (*du-huo*) 4

- Twelve-Ingredient Decoction with Rehmannia (*Ship-e-mi-ji-hwang Tang/ Shi-er-wei-di-huang Tang*):

  cooked rehmannia (*shu-di-huang*) 16, cornus (*shan-zhu-yu*) 8, poria (*fu-ling*) 6, alismatis (*ze-xie*) 6, moutan (*mu-dan-pi*) 4, lycium peel (*di-gu-pi*) 4, scrophularia (*xuan-shen*) 4, lycium fruit (*gou-qi-zi*) 4, raspberry (*fu-pen-zi*) 4, plantain (*che-qian-zi*) 4, schizonepeta (*jing-jie*) 4, sileris (*fang-feng*) 4

Tae-eumin Formulas

I. Exterior Diseases

A. Spine/Back Exterior Syndrome

1) Lumbar Vertebra Exterior Disease

- Ephedra Decoction to Release the Exterior (*Ma-hwang-bal-pyo Tang/ Ma-huang-fa-biao Tang*):

  platycodon (*jie-geng*) 12, ephedra (*ma-huang*) 6, ophiopogon (*mai-men-dong*) 4, scutellaria (*huang-qin*) 4, apricot seed (*xing-ren*) 4

2) Extreme Cold Syndrome

- Bear Gallbladder Powder (*Woong-dam San/ Xiong-dan San*): bear gallbladder (*xiong-dan*) 1.2-2

- Greater Cold and Lesser Heat Decoction (*Han-da-yeol-so Tang/ Han- duo-re-shao Tang*):

  coix (*yi-yi-ren*) 12, radish seed (radish seed (*lai-fu-zi*) 8, ophiopogon (*mai-men-dong*) 4, platycodon (*jie-geng*) 4, scutellaria (*huang-qin*) 4, apricot seed (*xing-ren*) 4, ephedra (*ma-huang*) 4, chestnut (*gan-li*) 7 pieces

B. Esophagus Cold Syndrome

1) Esophagus Cold Syndrome

- *Tae-eum* Regulate the Stomach Decoction (*Tae-eum-jo-wi Tang/ Tai-yin-tiao-wei Tang*):

  coix (*yi-yi-ren*) 12, chestnut (*gan-li*) 12, radish seed (*lai-fu-zi*) 8, schizandra (*wu-wei-zi*) 4, ophiopogon (*mai-men-dong*) 4, acorus (*shi-chang-pu*) 4, platycodon (*jie-geng*) 4, ephedra (*ma-huang*) 4

- Regulate the Stomach and Raise the Clear Decoction (*Jo-wi-seung-chung Tang/ Tiao-wei-sheng-qing Tang*):

  coix (*yi-yi-ren*) 12, chestnut (*gan-li*) 12, radish seed (*lai-fu-zi*) 6, ephedra (*ma-huang*) 4, platycodon (*jie-geng*) 4, ophiopogon (*mai-men-dong*) 4, schizandra (*wu-wei-zi*) 4, acorus (*shi-chang-pu*) 4, polygala (*yuan-zhi*) 4, asparagus (*tian-men-dong*) 4, zizyphus (*suan-zao-ren*) 4, longan fruit (*long-yan-rou*) 4

2) Convalescence

- Tonify the Lung Source Decoction (*Bo-pye-won Tang/ Bu-fei-yuan Tang*):

  ophiopogon (*mai-men-dong*) 12, platycodon (*jie-geng*) 8, schizandra (*wu-wei-zi*) 4

3) Asthma

- Stop the Asthma Decoction with Ephedra (*Ma-hwang-jung-chun Tang/ Ma-huang-ding-chuan Tang*):

  ephedra (*ma-huang*) 12, apricot seed (*xing-ren*) 6, scutellaria (*huang-qin*) 4, radish seed (*lai-fu-zi*) 4, mulberry bark (*sang-bai-pi*) 4, platycodon (*jie-geng*) 4, ophiopogon (*mai-men-dong*) 4, coltsfoot flower (*kuan-dong-hua*) 4, gingko (*bai-guo*) 21 pieces

4) Chest & Abdominal Pain

- Stop the Pain Decoction with Ephedra (*Ma-hwang-jung-tong Tang/ Ma-huang-ding-tong Tang*):

  coix (*yi-yi-ren*) 12, ephedra (*ma-huang*) 8, radish seed (*lai-fu-zi*) 8, apricot seed (*xing-ren*) 4, acorus (*shi-chang-pu*) 4, platycodon (*jie-geng*) 4, ophiopogon (*mai-men-dong*) 4, schizandra (*wu-wei-zi*) 4, longan (*long-yan-rou*) 4, biota (*bai-zi-ren*) 4, chestnut (*gan-li*) 7 pieces acanthopanax (*wu-jia-pi*) 4, pine flower (*song-hua*) 4, bran (*chu-tou-tang*) 4

The Answer Sheet to the Questionnaire for the Sasang Classification

For questions one to 15, fill out the correct answer number, and from question 16 on, check or circle the ones that relate to you.

1	2	3	4	5	6	7	8	9	10	11	12	13	14	15

16	17	18	19	20	21	22	23	24	25
26	27	28	29	30	31	32	33	34	35
36	37	38	39	40	41	42	43	44	45
46	47	48	49	50	51	52	53	54	55
56	57	58	59	60	61	62	63	64	65
66	67	68	69	70	71	72	73	74	75
76	77	78	79	80	81	82	83	84	85
86	87	88	89	90	91	92	93	94	95
96	97	98	99	100	101	102	103	104	105
106	107	108	109	110	111	112	113	114	115
116	117	118	119	120	121				

The Answer Key to the Questionnaire for the Sasang Classification

A. *Taeyangin*
1. ① 3. ① 6. ④ 7. ③ 7. ④ 8. ② 9. ④ 12. ①
17. 34. 40. 41. 48. 61. 62. 68. 78. 83. 90. 92. 97.
102. 108. 113.

B. *Soyangin*
1. ② 3. ① 4. ② 5. ③ 6. ② 7. ① 7. ④ 8. ①
9. ③ 10. ③ 12. ② 14. ② 15. ②
16. 18. 19. 20. 25. 26. 28. 31. 37. 39. 48. 49. 52.
54. 55. 57. 58. 59. 61. 63. 66. 69. 74. 75. 75. 84. 93.

C. *Tae-eumin*
1. ① 2. ① 3. ① 4. ③ 5. ① 6. ① 7. ③ 7. ④
8. ② 9. ① 10. ① 12. ① 13. ① 14. ① 15. ①

16. 21. 24. 26. 30. 39. 44. 45. 47. 48. 50. 53. 61.
73. 74. 76. 85. 88. 94. 103. 110. 117. 118. 121.

D. *Soeumin*
1. ③ 2. ③ 3. ② 4. ④ 5. ② 6. ② 7. ① 7. ②
8. ① 9. ② 10. ② 12. ④
22. 23. 24. 27. 29. 30. 33. 37. 38. 46. 47. 49. 50.
51. 52. 53. 56. 57. 59. 65. 66. 72. 73. 76. 77. 81.
84. 87. 89. 95. 96. 100. 101. 105. 111. 112. 114. 116.
120

Glossary

Activity-mind-body-matter. These four elements are the quaternary paradigm upon which Sasang philosophy is based. Dr. Lee Je-ma defined these as the four constituent elements that make up the universe and nature. They are divided into human components (body and mind) and nature/universe components (matter and activity).

Channels. Also known as meridians, the channels form a network of conduits or pathways through which vital energy (*qi*) circulates. Although there is no anatomical equivalent, the channels energetically connect various tissues, organs, and systems of the body. The human body consists of six basic channels, Taiyang, Yangming, Shaoyang, Taiyin, Shaoyin, and Jueyin. These are further subdivided into 12 principle channels depending on whether they belong to hand or foot channels.

Confucius (551-479 BC). Confucius is the most famous philosopher in the world and the most revered teacher in China and the Far East. He is known to have traveled widely through war torn China with his many followers preaching the virtues of benevolence and righteousness. He is also known to have written the commentaries on the *I Ching or Book of Changes*.

Confucianism. Confucianism, together with Buddhism and Taoism, is one of the major religions/philosophies of the East. It holds benevolence and righteousness to be characteristics of great importance. While Taoism focuses primarily on the patterns of nature, Confucianism is a more humanity-oriented philosophy. Dr. Lee Je-ma's teachings and his creation of Sasang Constitutional Medicine were primarily based upon Confucianist philosophies.

Constitution. Constitution, also referred to as body type, describes the nature of the body and mind that is innate and does not change over time. It refers to the hereditary factors that determine one's physical and mental characteristics as well as one's predisposition to illnesses. In Sasang Constitutional Medicine, people are classified into four basic types: *Soeumin, Soyangin, Tae-eumin,* and *Taeyangin,* based on the sizes of their internal organs.

Four Pillars. Astrological information such as the time, date, month and year of one's birth that is used in astrology, fortune telling and is even applied in medicine to check the condition of one's health.

Four Principles. This term was originally derived from Mencius. In Sasang Constitutional Medicine, the Four Principles refer to the four corners or four foundations of the constitutions. The Four Principles of the body refer to the size differences of the four organs (Lungs, Spleen, Liver, and Kidneys) that determine the constitution. The Four Principles of the mind refer to the original nature of benevolence, righteousness, propriety and wisdom or the four desires of rudeness, superficiality, greed, and indolence.

Constitutional Disease Syndrome. In *Longevity and Life Preservation in Eastern Medicine*, Dr. Lee Je-ma stated that human beings are born with different sized organs. This size distinction leads to the various disease states of each constitution. When the function of the larger organ becomes stronger while the smaller organ becomes weaker illness occurs. In *Soeumins*, the constitutional disease syndromes are divided into *Exterior Febrile Disease induced from the Kidney affected by Heat and Interior Cold Disease induced from the Stomach affected by Cold.* In *Soyangins*, they are divided into *Exterior Cold Disease induced from the Spleen affected by Cold and Interior Febrile Disease induced from the Stomach affected by Heat.* In *Tae-eumins,* they are divided into *Exterior Cold Disease induced from the Esophagus affected by Cold* and *Interior Febrile Disease induced from the Liver affected by Heat.* And finally in *Taeyangins*, they are divided into *Lumbar Vertebrae Disease induced by Exopathogen and Small Intestine Disease induced by Endopathogen.*

Four Burners. These are the four regions of the body (Upper Burner, Upper-Middle Burner, Lower-Middle Burner, and Lower Burner) that are associated with the functions of the organs. The burners are specific regions of the body and the organs involved in the various metabolic processes of the body. For instance, the Upper Burner is related to the Lungs and their energetic dispersing *qi* and fluids, while the Lower Burner is related to the Kidneys and their actions of releasing the food and water.

Eight Principles. This is the main diagnostic paradigm used in Syndrome Medicine to differentiate a syndrome. The Eight Principles consist of four categories with polar relationships, cold-hot, excess-deficiency, internal-external, and *yin-yang*. Hot-cold refers to the nature of a disease, while excess-deficiency denotes the strength of the body's resistance relative to the pathogenic force. Internal-external represents the location of the disease while *yin-yang* categorizes the disease. In clinical practice, hot-cold and excess-deficiency are the most important criteria of pathogenic differentiation and are vital to determining the proper course of treatment.

Emotions. The four basic emotions referred to in Sasang Constitutional Medicine (SCM) are sorrow, anger, joy and pleasure. These four emotions relate to the four organs and each emotion induces a different movement in the body. The sizes of the organs result from the varying degrees of the four emotions. In addition to the four emotions mentioned above, emotions in SCM also refer to specific behavioral tendencies of the individual constitutions, such as excessive masculinity in *Taeyangins*, excessive focus on external affairs in *Soyangins*, excessive focus on domestic affairs in *Tae-eumins*, and excessive femininity in *Soeumins.* Health and longevity result when there is harmony between the four emotions, while disease results from the reckless and violent expression of any of these emotions. In SCM, maintaining the proper emotional control is the most important ingredient to health and longevity.

Essence (*Jing*). *Jing*, the most refined and vital bodily substance, is stored in the Kidneys. It is responsible for birth, growth, aging and disease processes. In Sasang Constitutional Medicine, the essence is related to the mouth, the ability to taste, *Ye* (thick fluids), and the Lower Burner.

Five Blessings. The Five Blessings are discussed in Dr. Lee Je-ma's book, The New Edition on the Salvation of People. According to Dr. Lee Je-ma, the Five Blessings are the five things people should value most in their lives: longevity, a virtuous mind, desire for reading, building family wealth, and following through with one's plan in the world.

Five-Element Theory. The Five-Element Theory, also referred to as the Five-Phase Theory, is a system of correspondence that attempts to explain all phenomena and matter and their interactions with the five elements of wood, fire, earth, metal, and water. The five elements correspond with colors, sounds, seasons, directions, weather, organs, emotions, etc. The theory also describes cycles of generation and control while using these cycles to explain the functional relationships and the various processes of the natural world. The generating cycle describes the following processes: wood generates fire, fire generates earth, earth generates metal, and metal generates water. The controlling cycle describes the following processes: wood controls earth, earth controls water, water controls fire, fire controls metal, and metal controls wood. This theory, together with the *yin-yang* Theory, is used extensively in traditional Syndrome Medicine.

Golden Mean. This is the most important principle of Confucianism. It is the "middle path" that all followers of Confucianism attempt to attain and practice in their daily lives. Dr. Lee Je-ma based Sasang Constitutional Medicine on this concept.

I Ching. The *Book of Changes* is the oldest book in the world. In the West, it is commonly known as a book of divination, however, every aspect of Eastern culture from politics and economics to astronomy, astrology, and Eastern medicine is based upon the principles of this book, namely *yin* and *yang*.

Inner Classic (Nei Jing). Known as the *Yellow Emperor's Classic of Internal Medicine*, this 18-volume text is the oldest book describing the principles of Eastern medicine and is estimated to have been written circa 722 B.C. to 221 B.C. This classic is divided into two sections, the Su Wen (Simple Questions) and the Ling Shu (Spiritual Axis). The Su Wen discusses theories of anatomy, physiology, pathology, therapeutics and health cultivation. The Ling Shu discusses theories of acupuncture and moxibustion.

Lee Je-ma (1837-1900). A Confucianist and medical scholar of the later Chosun dynasty (1392-1910 AD), Dr. Lee Je-ma rebelled against the rampant abuse of Neo-Confucianism and created his own Sasang philosophy based upon ideals of Reformed Confucianism. He revolutionized Eastern medicine with his advent of Sasang Constitutional Theory, which uses hereditary factors to diagnose, treat, and prevent illnesses. He wrote three books, *Longevity and Life Preservation in Eastern Medicine* (*Dong-ui susebowon*), *Manuscript of Science* (*Gyeokchigo*), and *The New Edition on the Salvation of People* (*Jaejungsinpyeon*).

Longevity and Life Preservation in Eastern Medicine (*Dong-ui susebowon*). This is the bible of Sasang Constitutional Medicine (SCM) and all of the basic principles of SCM are based upon this text. It was completed by Dr. Lee Je-ma in 1894 and is comprised of four volumes, which have two basic parts, basic theories and clinical studies. Along with the book *Manuscript of Science*, this book is the most typical of Dr. Lee Je-ma's work. It is used as the main text in all 11 colleges of Eastern medicine in Korea.

Manuscript of Science (*Gyeokchigo*). *Manuscript of Science* was completed by Dr. Lee Je-ma in 1893 after 14 years of work, and is comprised of three chapters: "The Summary of Confucianism," "Self-cultivation" and "Cautions on Insincerity." In this book, Dr. Lee Je-ma draws on teachings of ancient Confucianism rather than Neo-Confucianism. His other work, *Longevity and Life Preservation in Eastern Medicine* (*Dong-ui susebowon*), explains theories of Sasang Constitutional Medicine in his own humanized and practical philosophy, which came prior to his creation of the SCM.

Mencius (372-289 BC). The most famous Confucian scholar, Mencius is known for his keynote theory of the "innate goodness" of human nature. He disseminated the teachings of Confucius, the basic virtue of benevolence, and advocated the Four Principles of benevolence, righteousness, propriety, and wisdom. Among all Confucian scholars, Dr. Lee Je-ma held Mencius in the highest esteem.

Nature. Nature refers to a person's innate nature and that which is bestowed by heaven. It is one's disposition, temperament, and constitution. In Sasang Constitutional Medicine, the *nature* of *Taeyangins* is described as "always rushing forward without looking back" and for *Soyangins* it is "always starting projects without organizing or completing them." The *nature* of *Tae-eumins* is "staying calm and disliking movements" and for *Soeumins* it is "staying home rather than going out."

Order. That which we receive from heaven. It is heaven's order or decree, our fate or destiny.

Pathogenic *Qi*. Indicates any force or entity either inside or outside the body that hinders normal physiological processes and creates pathological changes.

Neo-Confucianism. A more recent school of Confucianism that combines Confucianism with Taoism and Buddhism. It was begun circa the 11th century in the Song dynasty by Cheng Zi and Zhou Don I, and made popular by the most famous Neo-Confucianist, Zhu Xi.

Principles of *Li* and *Qi*. *Li* is the organizing principle or universal law, while *qi* is the manifestation or substantive aspect of all things. *Li* is the implicit principle that governs and causes all things to manifest. Neo-Confucianism regards the *li* as similar to *taichi* and *tao*.

***Qi*.** *Qi* is generally translated as life force, life energy, dynamic energy, or bio-energy. It is the fundamental force of nature that is the basis of all change and is associated with the creation or formation of all living entities. *Qi* also implies the manifestation of all phenomena and matter in the universe when compared to *li*, the organizing principle. Sasang Constitutional Medicine describes the movement of *qi* in two basic sets of four movements. One is dispersing, gathering, accumulating and releasing and the other is ascending, obliquely ascending, descending, and obliquely descending. These movements are intimately related to the organs, Burners, and emotions.

Righteous *Qi*. The Righteous *qi* is the vital energy that circulates in the channels. It nourishes, harmonizes and regulates various bodily processes and activities such as metabolism, immunity, and healing. It refers to three key factors, normal physiological processes, resistance against disease and the ability to recover from disease.

Sasang. Sasang is a term derived from the *I Ching*, and implies four symbols or images named *taeyang, soyang, tae-eum, and soeum* from which Dr. Lee Je-ma derived the names of the individual constitutions. In the context of Sasang philosophy, the foundation of Sasang Constitutional Medicine, Sasang implies activity, mind, body, and matter, the fundamental units of all phenomena and matter in the universe.

***Shang Han Lun* (Six Channel Disease Theory).** This theory considers febrile diseases caused by the cold. It discusses the diagnosis and treatment of febrile diseases according to the six channels, *taiyang* (Greater *yang*), *yangming* (Extreme *yang*), *shaoyang* (Lesser *yang*), *taiyin* (Greater *yin*), *shaoyin* (Lesser *yin*), and *jueyin* (Declining *yin*).

***Soeumin*.** One of the four constitutions of Sasang Constitutional Medicine, *Soeumins* have large Kidneys and a small Spleen. Physically, *Soeumins* have greater lower body development with well-developed hips. They are gentle and calm and easily form communal bonds. They are also meticulous and crafty. *Soeumins* are considered healthy when their digestion is sound.

***Soyangin*.** One of the four constitutions of Sasang Constitutional

Medicine, *Soyangins* have a large Spleen and small Kidneys. Physically, *Soyangins* have well-developed upper bodies with wide shoulders tapering down to narrow waist and hips. They are strong and quick, and are skilled in management and carrying forward with plans. *Soyangins* tend to harbor anxiety and are considered healthy when they have regular bowel movements.

Spirit (*Shen*). The *Shen* regulates life phenomena. It is a vital manifestation of human life and is expressed in the clarity and luminosity of a person's eyes and complexion, and in one's general expressions, reactions, and behaviors. Traditionally, it is said to be formed by a combination of vital energy (*qi*) and essence (*jing*). In Sasang Constitutional Medicine, the spirit is related to the ears and hearing, the brain, the Upper Burner, and Jin (thin and clear body fluids).

Syndrome Medicine. This is the TCM as it is well known. It is based on the differentiation of syndromes, a generalized summary of patient's signs and symptoms, as well as the location, nature, and cause of a disease. Furthermore, it addresses the dynamic relationship between pathogenic factors and the body's Righteous *qi*. This collective data is obtained according to theories of Eastern medicine and its diagnostic methods. Syndrome Medicine is based on *yin-yang* and the Five Element theories. It uses the principle of tonifying deficiency and sedating excess to balance the *yin* and *yang* of the body. Syndrome Medicine focuses on such environmental factors as stress and germs, while Sasang Constitutional Medicine focuses on hereditary factors or genetics.

Tae-eumin. One of the four constitutions of Sasang Constitutional Medicine, *Tae-eumins* have a large Liver and small Lungs. Physically, *Tae-eumins* have greater lower body than upper body development and thick waists. They are very patient and persistent and generally accomplish what they start. *Tae-eumins* tend to hold fear inside and are considered healthy if they are sweating well.

Taeyangin. One of the four constitutions of Sasang Constitutional

Medicine, *Taeyangins* have large Lungs and a small Liver. Physically, *Taeyangins* have greater upper body than lower body development with the broad chest and thick neck. They are great communicators when socializing and are resolute. *Taeyangins* tend to have urgent minds and quick temper. They are healthy when they have no problem with their urination.

Vast Flowing *Qi*. The vast flowing *qi* is moral courage devoid of shame. It is deeply rooted in morality and is exceedingly just and fair. According to Dr. Lee Je-ma, it is said to emerge from the Lungs, Spleen, Liver and Kidneys, when the *qi* of these four organs (benevolence, righteousness, propriety, and wisdom) is amplified.

Vast Flowing Principle. According to Dr. Lee Je-ma, the vast flowing principle is said to emerge from the Heart or the mind when the desires of the mind (rudeness, superficiality, greed, and indolence) are clearly distinguished.

***Wei* (Protective) *Qi*.** The vital energy responsible for maintaining the body temperature and providing resistance to pathogenic factors in the environment. It is said to flow in and out of acupuncture channels.

***Yin-Yang*.** The positive and negative forces of nature, these are polar, yet mutually interdependent forces that create and transform all phenomena. The theory of *yin* and *yang*, along with the theory of the Five Elements forms the foundation of Eastern medicine. In the human body, the proper balance of *yin* and *yang* is vital to maintaining health, while an imbalance of *yin* and *yang* results in disease.

Ying (Nutritive) *Qi*. As its name implies, this vital energy nourishes the tissues, organs, and systems of the body. It flows through the acupuncture channels and is an integral component of the blood.

Zhang Zhong-jing (142-220 AD). A distinguished medical scholar, Dr. Zhang Zhong-jing created the Shan Han Theory. In addition, he established the theory of eastern herbal prescriptions, invented treatment principles, and fathered the ideas of the "differentiation of syndromes" and the "discussion of treatments."

Zhu Xi (1130-1200 AD). A major figure in Chinese philosophy, Zhu Xi was one of the founders of Neo-Confucianism. He implemented a restructuring of Confucianism around the metaphysical principle of the *li* (universal organizing principle) and *qi* (manifestation/substance) thus transforming Confucianism.

Index

- SWEAT-36·65

About the Author and Translators

Song Il-byung OMD, Ph.D.

Professor Song Il-byung is currently the head professor of the Department of Sasang Constitutional Medicine at the prestigious Kyung Hee University in Korea. He is also the Chief Physician of Eastern medicine at the Kyung Hee University Medical Center. Professor Song has dedicated his life to studying, researching, and teaching Sasang Constitutional Medicine. He is currently the foremost exponent of this system of medicine in Korea. The heads of all ten Sasang Constitutional Medicine Departments of the other Eastern medical universities in Korea have, at one time, been students of Professor Song's.

He has written two other books, *The Textbook of Sasang Constitutional Medicine* and *A Beginner's Guide to Sasang Constitutional Medicine*, and has published numerous research papers and articles. He is the editor-in-chief of the *Journal of Sasang Constitutional Medicine* that is published twice a year in Korea.

He is currently on the President's Advisory Board on Eastern medicine and has formerly served as the President of the Society of Sasang Constitutional Medicine, a branch under the Association of Korean Oriental Medicine, which has over 3,000 members. He was also previously the president of the Society of the Korean Oriental Medical Center.

Joseph K. Kim, OMD, Ph.D.

As a third generation practitioner of Eastern medicine, Dr. Joseph K. Kim specializes in Sasang Constitutional Medicine. He has served as Chairman of the Department of Eastern Medicine at Emperor's College of Traditional Oriental Medicine in Los

Angeles, and is currently an acupuncture researcher at the University of California at Irvine, where he is studying the effects of acupuncture on brain patterns as translated by a functional MRI.

Dr. Kim received advanced clinical training in China and Korea and has three books in print. He translated and revised Cho Hun-young's *Oriental Medicine: A Modern Interpretation,* and has written *Compass of Health* and *Science and Tao of I Ching*. Additionally, he has published many articles about Eastern medicine.

Dr. Kim also has more than 20 years of martial arts training, including *qigong* and *taichi.* He served as the team doctor for the United States *Taekwondo* Team (ITF) of 1988. He maintains a private practice in Encino, California.

Huh Mahn-hoi, OMD, Ph.D.

OMD, Kyung Hee University
Ph.D. Kyung Hee University, Graduate School of Oriental Medicine
Professor of Kyung Won University
Doctor of Je Won Local Clinic*

---

*If you have any questions about SCM or in the contents of this book, please visit our website www.esasang.com
or e-mail us manwhi@hanmail.net